Smart Fitness Choices

Making Informed Decisions for a Healthier Lifestyle

Waldo Burrows

Smart Fitness Choices

clarifying purposes only and are owned by the owners themselves, not affiliated with this document.

Table of Contents

Chapter 1: Assessing Your Current Fitness Level

Conducting a Fitness Self-Assessment

Taking the first step in a fitness journey involves understanding your starting point, and conducting a fitness self-assessment is an invaluable tool in this process. Knowing your current fitness level helps tailor a program that meets your specific needs and goals, ensuring safety and effectiveness. Let's explore the key components of a comprehensive fitness self-assessment and how you can use the results to create a customized fitness plan.

Start with assessing your cardiovascular endurance. This can be done through a simple test like the three-minute step test, which measures how quickly your heart rate returns to normal after exercise. Find a sturdy step or platform about 12 inches high. Step up and down at a consistent pace for three minutes, then sit down and measure your heart rate for one full minute. Compare your recovery heart rate to standard norms for your age and gender. This will give you an idea of your cardiovascular fitness level and help set a baseline for improvement.

Next, evaluate your muscular strength and endurance. One way to measure upper body strength is through a push-up test. Perform as many push-ups as you can with proper form until you can no longer maintain it. Keep track of the number you complete. For lower body strength, the wall sit test is effective. Sit against a wall with your knees at a right angle and hold the position as long as possible. Record the duration you can maintain the position. These tests provide insights into your muscular endurance and highlight areas needing focus in your training program.

Flexibility is another crucial aspect of fitness. The sit-and-reach test is a common method to assess the flexibility of your lower back and hamstrings. Sit on the floor with your legs straight out in front of you, feet flat against a box or wall. Slowly reach forward as far as you can without bending your knees, and measure the distance between your fingertips and your feet. Improving flexibility can enhance overall movement efficiency and reduce the risk of injury, so it's important to understand your starting point.

Body composition analysis provides a clearer picture of your overall health. While body weight alone doesn't account for muscle mass, fat distribution, and bone density, body composition analysis does. Tools like bioelectrical impedance scales, skinfold calipers, or even professional assessments like DEXA scans can help determine your body fat percentage. Understanding your body composition helps set realistic goals, whether it's losing fat, gaining muscle, or maintaining your current state while improving other fitness aspects.

Balance is often overlooked but is essential for overall fitness and injury prevention. A simple balance test is the one-leg stand. Stand on one leg with your eyes closed and time how long you can maintain your balance without putting your foot down or opening your eyes. Test both legs, and note the differences. Balance exercises can be integrated into your fitness routine, especially if you find this area needs improvement.

Monitoring resting heart rate (RHR) provides insights into your cardiovascular health. Measure your pulse first thing in the morning before getting out of bed. A lower RHR typically indicates a higher level of cardiovascular fitness. Track your RHR over time to see how it changes with your fitness improvements.

A fitness self-assessment also includes identifying any physical limitations or past injuries. Note any pain or discomfort during exercises, which can indicate underlying issues that need addressing before starting an intense fitness regimen. Consulting with a healthcare professional or physical therapist can provide a more thorough assessment and guidance on accommodating any limitations in your workout plan.

Once you've gathered all this data, it's time to interpret the results and set SMART goals. For example, if your cardiovascular endurance is below average, you might set a goal to improve your step test performance by a certain number of beats per minute within the next three months. If your upper body strength is lacking, you could aim to increase your push-up count by 20% over the same period.

Creating a balanced workout plan based on your assessment results is the next step. This plan should include cardiovascular exercises, strength training, flexibility exercises, and balance training. For instance, if your flexibility is limited, incorporate stretching or yoga sessions into your weekly routine. If your muscular endurance needs improvement, include both upper and lower body strength training exercises several times a week.

It's important to periodically re-assess your fitness levels to track progress and adjust your workout plan as needed. Every six to eight weeks, repeat the same assessments to see how far you've come and identify new areas for improvement. This ongoing evaluation helps keep you motivated and ensures your fitness program evolves with your changing fitness levels.

Consider the story of Alex, who began his fitness journey with a comprehensive self-assessment. Alex found his cardiovascular endurance was below average, his upper body strength was adequate, but his flexibility and balance were poor. By setting specific, achievable goals and creating a balanced workout plan focusing on these areas, Alex made significant progress. After six weeks, his step test results improved markedly, his push-up count increased, and he could reach further in the sit-and-reach test. His balance also improved, allowing him to stand on one leg much longer than before.

Alex's experience highlights the importance of a fitness self-assessment in providing a clear starting point and direction for your fitness journey. It ensures your efforts are targeted and effective, maximizing your progress and minimizing the risk of injury. By regularly re-assessing and adjusting your plan, you stay on track and continuously challenge yourself to achieve new fitness milestones.

In conclusion, conducting a fitness self-assessment is a crucial first step in any fitness program. It provides a clear picture of your current fitness level, helps set realistic goals, and informs the creation of a personalized workout plan. By focusing on all aspects of fitness—cardiovascular endurance, muscular strength and endurance, flexibility, body composition, and balance—you ensure a comprehensive approach that leads to sustainable, long-term improvements in your health and well-being.

Understanding Your Body Composition

Understanding your body composition is vital to creating a sustainable and effective fitness plan. Body composition refers to the percentages of fat, bone, water, and muscle in your body. Unlike body weight alone, which doesn't differentiate between these components, body composition provides a clearer picture of your overall health and fitness. Knowing the makeup of your body helps in setting realistic goals, tracking progress, and tailoring your exercise and nutrition plans to meet your specific needs.

Body composition can be divided into two main categories: fat mass and fat-free mass. Fat mass includes all the fat tissue in your body, while fat-free mass is composed of muscles, bones, water, and organs. Understanding the balance between these two components is crucial for evaluating your health. High levels of body fat, especially visceral fat stored around internal organs, can increase the risk of chronic diseases like heart disease, diabetes, and certain cancers. On the other hand, maintaining a healthy proportion of muscle mass is essential for strength, mobility, and metabolic health.

To accurately assess body composition, several methods are available, each with its own advantages and limitations. One of the most accessible methods is the use of skinfold calipers, which measure the thickness of subcutaneous fat at specific body sites. This method requires some skill and consistency to ensure accurate measurements. Typically, skinfold measurements are taken at the triceps, biceps, subscapular (below the shoulder blade), and suprailiac (above the hip bone) regions. These measurements are then used in equations to estimate body fat percentage. While not the most precise method, it provides a useful baseline for tracking changes over time.

Bioelectrical impedance analysis (BIA) is another common method. BIA devices send a small electrical current through the body and measure the resistance to the current flow. Since muscle tissue conducts electricity better than fat tissue, the device can estimate body composition based on the resistance encountered. BIA is quick and non-invasive, but its accuracy can be affected by factors such as hydration status, meal timing, and exercise. For more reliable results, it's best to follow the manufacturer's guidelines regarding preparation and consistency.

For those seeking more precise measurements, dual-energy X-ray absorptiometry (DEXA) scans and hydrostatic weighing are considered gold standards. DEXA scans use low-dose X-rays to differentiate between bone mass, lean mass, and fat mass, providing a detailed picture of body composition. This method is highly accurate but also more expensive and less accessible. Hydrostatic weighing, often available at universities or specialized facilities, involves being weighed underwater. Since fat tissue is less dense than water, this method can determine body density and, subsequently, body composition. While extremely accurate, it is also more time-consuming and less convenient than other methods.

Regardless of the method used, interpreting the results is key to understanding your body composition. For example, a body fat percentage of 15-20% is generally considered healthy for men, while 20-25% is typical for women. These ranges can vary depending on age, fitness level, and individual goals. Athletes, for instance, often have lower body fat percentages due to higher muscle mass and rigorous training regimens.

Once you have a clear understanding of your body composition, setting realistic and achievable goals becomes more straightforward. If the goal is fat loss, focus on creating a calorie deficit through a combination of diet and exercise. Incorporate both aerobic exercises, such as running or cycling, and strength training to preserve muscle mass while reducing fat. Remember, rapid weight loss often results in muscle loss as well, so aim for a gradual reduction of 1-2 pounds per week.

Building muscle, on the other hand, requires a calorie surplus and a focus on resistance training. Compound exercises like squats, deadlifts, and bench presses are particularly effective for stimulating muscle growth. Ensure that your diet includes sufficient protein, typically around 1.2 to 2.2 grams per kilogram of body weight, to support muscle repair and growth. Monitor your progress by regularly reassessing your body composition and adjusting your training and nutrition plans as needed.

Hydration and sleep also play vital roles in body composition. Drinking adequate water helps maintain muscle function and metabolic processes, while proper sleep is crucial for recovery and hormonal balance. Aim for at least 8 glasses of water per day and 7-9 hours of quality sleep each night to support your fitness goals.

Tracking progress is essential for staying motivated and making informed adjustments to your fitness plan. Regularly measure your body composition, but avoid obsessing over daily fluctuations. Instead, focus on long-term trends and how you feel overall. Keep a journal or use a fitness app to log your measurements, workouts, and dietary habits. This information can provide valuable insights into what works best for your body and help you stay on track.

Consider the story of John, a 35-year-old office worker who decided to improve his health after years of sedentary living. Initially, John focused solely on losing weight, but after a few months, he hit a plateau and felt frustrated. Upon assessing his body composition, he realized that while he had lost some fat, he also lost muscle mass. This insight prompted John to shift his focus to strength training and a balanced diet rich in protein. Over time, his body composition improved significantly, with a reduction in fat mass and an increase in lean muscle. John felt stronger, more energetic, and better equipped to handle daily activities.

John's journey highlights the importance of understanding body composition beyond just weight loss. By focusing on the balance of fat and muscle, you can achieve a healthier and more sustainable transformation. Remember, the goal is to improve overall health, not just to change the number on the scale.

In summary, understanding your body composition is a fundamental aspect of any fitness journey. By measuring and interpreting your body fat percentage, muscle mass, and other components, you gain valuable insights into your health and fitness. Use this information to set realistic goals, tailor your exercise and nutrition plans, and track your progress over time. Prioritizing body composition over mere weight loss leads to a more balanced, healthier, and sustainable approach to fitness. Embrace this knowledge and take control of your fitness journey, focusing on long-term health and well-being.

Evaluating Your Cardiovascular Health

Understanding and evaluating your cardiovascular health is a critical step in establishing a solid foundation for your fitness journey. Cardiovascular health encompasses the efficiency and capacity of your heart, lungs, and circulatory system to supply oxygen-rich blood to your muscles during sustained physical activity. This chapter will guide you through the importance of cardiovascular health, how to assess it effectively, and how to use this information to tailor your fitness goals.

Imagine you are preparing to embark on a challenging hike. You wouldn't set off without first checking the condition of your gear, ensuring you have the right supplies, and understanding the terrain ahead. Similarly, before diving into a fitness regimen, it's essential to evaluate your cardiovascular health to navigate your journey safely and effectively.

Begin by measuring your resting heart rate (RHR), an easy and informative indicator of cardiovascular fitness. Your RHR is the number of times your heart beats per minute while at rest. Typically, a lower RHR signifies a more efficient heart function and better cardiovascular fitness. To measure your RHR, find a quiet place and sit or lie down. Use your index and middle fingers to locate your pulse on your wrist or neck, count the beats for 60 seconds, and record the number. Repeat this process on different days at the same time to get an accurate average. For most adults, a normal RHR ranges from 60 to 100 beats per minute, with athletes often having RHRs as low as 40 beats per minute.

Next, consider the step test, a simple yet effective method to evaluate your cardiovascular endurance. For this test, you'll need a 12-inch step and a stopwatch. Step up and down at a consistent pace for three minutes, then immediately sit down and measure your heart rate for one minute. The quicker your heart rate returns to normal, the better your cardiovascular fitness. Compare your results with standard recovery heart rate charts to determine your fitness level. This test provides a practical baseline to monitor improvements over time.

Another valuable assessment is the Cooper 12-minute run test, which measures how far you can run or walk in twelve minutes. This test requires a flat, measured track and a stopwatch. Warm up thoroughly, then run or walk as far as possible in twelve minutes. Record the distance covered and compare it to normative data for your age and gender. This test not only gauges your cardiovascular endurance but also helps set realistic goals for improvement.

The VO2 max test is considered the gold standard for assessing cardiovascular fitness. VO2 max represents the maximum amount of oxygen your body can utilize during intense exercise. While this test is typically performed in a lab setting using specialized equipment, there are field tests and estimations available. One popular method is the Rockport walking test. Walk one mile as quickly as possible on a flat surface, then measure your heart rate at the end. Use a VO2 max calculator, which takes into account your weight, age, gender, time taken, and heart rate, to estimate your VO2 max. Higher VO2 max values indicate superior cardiovascular fitness.

Blood pressure is another critical component of cardiovascular health. High blood pressure, or hypertension, can lead to serious health complications like heart disease and stroke. Regular monitoring of your blood pressure provides insights into your cardiovascular health and helps identify potential issues early. A normal blood pressure reading is generally considered to be around 120/80 mm Hg. If your readings are consistently above this range, it's advisable to consult a healthcare professional for further evaluation and management.

In addition to these physical tests, lifestyle factors play a significant role in cardiovascular health. Assess your diet, physical activity levels, smoking status, and stress levels. A diet rich in fruits, vegetables, whole grains, lean proteins, and healthy fats supports heart health. Regular physical activity, at least 150 minutes of moderate-intensity or 75 minutes of high-intensity exercise per week, is crucial. Avoid smoking, as it significantly damages cardiovascular health, and find effective stress management techniques such as mindfulness, yoga, or hobbies you enjoy.

Armed with the results of these assessments, you can create a personalized fitness plan tailored to your cardiovascular health. For instance, if your RHR is on the higher side, incorporating more aerobic activities like brisk walking, cycling, or swimming can help lower it over time. If your step test recovery heart rate is slower than average, gradually increasing the intensity and duration of your cardio workouts will improve your endurance. If your VO2 max is lower than expected, interval training, which alternates between high and low-intensity exercise, can effectively boost your aerobic capacity.

Tracking your progress is essential. Keep a fitness journal or use a digital app to log your RHR, step test results, Cooper test distances, VO2 max estimates, and blood pressure readings. Regularly reviewing these metrics helps you stay motivated and adjust your fitness plan as needed. For example, if you notice your RHR decreasing and your step test recovery improving, you're on the right track. If progress stalls, consider tweaking your routine by adding variety or consulting a fitness professional for advice.

Personal stories often illuminate the journey. Take Sarah, a 45-year-old office worker who decided to improve her health after a routine check-up revealed high blood pressure and a high RHR. Sarah began with a thorough cardiovascular assessment, discovering her endurance was below average. She started a tailored program focusing on brisk walking and gradually incorporated jogging and interval training. Over six months, Sarah's RHR decreased, her blood pressure normalized, and she felt more energetic and positive. Her story underscores the transformative power of understanding and improving cardiovascular health.

Incorporating cardiovascular health evaluations into your fitness journey ensures a targeted and effective approach. It allows you to identify strengths and weaknesses, set realistic goals, and monitor progress accurately. Remember, the heart is the engine that drives your fitness journey. Keeping it strong and healthy is paramount to achieving long-term success and overall well-being.

In conclusion, evaluating your cardiovascular health is a foundational step in crafting a successful fitness plan. Through methods like resting heart rate measurement, step tests, the Cooper 12-minute run, VO2 max estimations, and regular blood pressure monitoring, you gain a comprehensive understanding of your cardiovascular fitness. Coupled with healthy lifestyle choices and consistent tracking, these assessments empower you to make informed decisions and achieve your fitness goals. Prioritize your heart health, and you'll pave the way for a more energized, resilient, and fulfilling life.

Flexibility and Mobility Tests

Flexibility and mobility are crucial components of overall fitness and significantly impact your performance in various physical activities. They contribute to the efficiency and safety of your movements, reduce the risk of injury, and enhance your ability to perform daily tasks. Understanding your current level of flexibility and mobility through specific tests can help you identify areas for improvement and tailor your fitness routine accordingly.

Flexibility refers to the ability of your muscles and other soft tissues to stretch and allow a joint to move through its full range of motion. Mobility, on the other hand, involves the ability of a joint to move freely through its range of motion, encompassing flexibility but also including the strength, coordination, and control required for movement. Both are essential for maintaining functional fitness and preventing injuries.

One of the most common tests for evaluating flexibility is the sit-and-reach test. This simple test assesses the flexibility of your lower back and hamstring muscles. To perform the sit-and-reach test, sit on the floor with your legs extended straight in front of you, feet against a box or wall, and knees flat. Place one hand on top of the other and slowly reach forward as far as possible without bouncing, holding the position for a few seconds. Measure the distance from your toes to the tips of your fingers. If you can reach beyond your toes, you have good flexibility in this area. If you fall short, you might need to incorporate more stretching exercises for your lower back and hamstrings into your routine.

Another useful flexibility test is the shoulder flexibility test, which assesses the range of motion in your shoulder joints. Stand tall and extend one arm straight up, then bend your elbow and reach down behind your head. Simultaneously, extend the other arm down and behind your back, reaching up towards the other hand. Try to touch your fingertips together. If you can touch or overlap your fingers, you have good shoulder flexibility. If not, you may need to work on stretching and strengthening your shoulder muscles.

The Thomas test is an effective way to evaluate the flexibility of your hip flexors. Lie on your back on a flat surface, pull one knee towards your chest and hold it with both hands. Allow the other leg to relax and extend down towards the floor. If the extended leg remains flat on the surface without lifting, you have adequate hip flexor flexibility. If it lifts off the surface, it indicates tight hip flexors, which can affect your posture and contribute to lower back pain.

Assessing your mobility is equally important. The overhead squat test is a comprehensive test that evaluates the mobility of your ankles, knees, hips, shoulders, and thoracic spine. Stand with your feet shoulder-width apart and hold a broomstick or dowel overhead with your arms fully extended. Perform a squat, keeping the dowel overhead and your heels flat on the ground. Ideally, you should be able to squat down until your thighs are parallel to the floor without the dowel moving forward or your heels lifting. If you struggle with this movement, it can indicate mobility restrictions in various joints, requiring targeted exercises to address these limitations.

The ankle mobility test helps evaluate the flexibility and range of motion in your ankle joints. Stand facing a wall with your toes about 4 inches away. Keeping your heel on the floor, bend your knee and try to touch it to the wall. If you can do this without lifting your heel, you have good ankle mobility. Limited ankle mobility can affect your performance in activities like running, jumping, and squatting, so it's important to address any restrictions through stretching and strengthening exercises.

Hip mobility is crucial for various movements, including running, jumping, and squatting. The 90/90 stretch test is a good way to assess your hip mobility. Sit on the floor with one leg bent at a 90-degree angle in front of you and the other leg bent at a 90-degree angle behind you. Lean forward over the front leg, keeping your back straight. A significant restriction in your ability to lean forward indicates tightness in your hip muscles. Repeat on the other side to compare flexibility between both hips.

Incorporating regular flexibility and mobility exercises into your fitness routine can improve your performance and reduce the risk of injuries. Dynamic stretching, which involves moving parts of your body and gradually increasing reach, speed, or both, is effective before workouts. Examples include leg swings, arm circles, and torso twists. These movements help increase blood flow and prepare your muscles for exercise.

Static stretching, where you hold a stretch for 15-60 seconds, is more effective post-workout. It helps lengthen muscles that have been tightened during exercise. Examples include hamstring stretches, quadriceps stretches, and chest stretches. Focus on breathing deeply and relaxing into each stretch to maximize its effectiveness.

Foam rolling is another useful technique for improving flexibility and mobility. It involves using a foam roller to apply pressure to tight muscles and fascia, the connective tissue surrounding muscles. This self-myofascial release technique helps break up scar tissue and adhesions, improving muscle elasticity and joint range of motion. Roll slowly over each muscle group, pausing on any tender spots for 20-30 seconds.

Yoga and Pilates are excellent for enhancing flexibility and mobility. Both practices emphasize controlled movements, balance, and strength, which contribute to improved range of motion and overall body awareness. Incorporating yoga or Pilates sessions into your weekly routine can provide significant benefits for your flexibility and mobility.

Consider the story of Emily, a 28-year-old office worker who often experienced lower back pain and stiffness. After performing the sit-and-reach test, she realized her hamstring flexibility was limited. Emily decided to integrate daily hamstring stretches and weekly yoga sessions into her routine. Over a few months, her flexibility improved, and her back pain diminished. She also noticed enhanced performance in her other workouts, thanks to her increased range of motion.

Emily's experience highlights the importance of regularly assessing and addressing flexibility and mobility. By understanding your current abilities and incorporating targeted exercises, you can enhance your overall fitness and reduce the risk of injuries. Remember, flexibility and mobility are not static; they can improve with consistent effort and attention.

In summary, flexibility and mobility tests are essential tools for evaluating your current fitness level and identifying areas for improvement. By incorporating dynamic and static stretches, foam rolling, and practices like yoga or Pilates, you can enhance your flexibility and mobility, leading to better performance and reduced injury risk. Regularly assess your progress and adjust your routine as needed to maintain and improve your range of motion. Embrace the journey towards greater flexibility and mobility, and enjoy the benefits of a more functional and resilient body.

Setting a Baseline for Progress

Establishing a baseline is a fundamental step in any fitness journey. It serves as a starting point from which you can measure progress, set realistic goals, and tailor your exercise regimen to meet your specific needs. Without a baseline, it's challenging to gauge improvements or identify areas that require additional focus. This chapter delves into the importance of setting a baseline, the methods to do so, and how to use this information to enhance your fitness journey.

When embarking on a fitness program, it's essential to understand your current physical condition. This involves assessing various aspects of fitness, including cardiovascular endurance, muscular strength and endurance, flexibility, and body composition. By evaluating these components, you can create a comprehensive picture of your health and fitness level.

One of the most effective ways to assess cardiovascular endurance is through the use of aerobic fitness tests. The most common and accessible test is the 12-minute run or walk test, also known as the Cooper Test. In this test, you aim to cover as much distance as possible in 12 minutes. The distance you cover is then compared to normative data, which categorizes your cardiovascular fitness level. This test provides a clear metric that can be re-evaluated periodically to track improvements in cardiovascular endurance.

Muscular strength can be assessed through various exercises that target different muscle groups. For example, the one-repetition maximum (1RM) test is commonly used to measure the maximal amount of weight a person can lift in a single repetition for a given exercise, such as the bench press or squat. However, for beginners or those without access to heavy weights, alternative tests like the push-up or plank tests can be used. The push-up test measures upper body strength and endurance by counting the number of push-ups you can perform without rest. Similarly, the plank test measures core strength by timing how long you can hold a plank position. These tests provide valuable benchmarks that can be used to track progress over time.

Flexibility is another critical component of fitness that can be assessed using various tests. The sit-and-reach test, mentioned in the previous chapter, is a simple and effective way to measure the flexibility of your lower back and hamstrings. Additionally, the shoulder flexibility test can help assess the range of motion in your shoulders. These tests are essential for identifying tight areas that may need targeted stretching and mobility exercises.

Body composition, which refers to the proportion of fat and non-fat mass in your body, is a crucial aspect of overall fitness. Several methods can be used to assess body composition, ranging from simple techniques like body mass index (BMI) calculations to more advanced methods like bioelectrical impedance analysis (BIA) or dual-energy X-ray absorptiometry (DEXA) scans. While BMI provides a general indication of whether you are underweight, normal weight, overweight, or obese, it does not differentiate between muscle and fat mass. Therefore, methods like BIA or DEXA, which provide a more detailed breakdown of body composition, are preferable if available.

Once you have established your baseline through these assessments, the next step is to set realistic and specific goals. Goals should be SMART: Specific, Measurable, Achievable, Relevant, and Time-bound. For example, instead of setting a vague goal like "get in shape," a SMART goal would be "increase my 12-minute run distance by 10% over the next three months." This goal is specific (increase run distance), measurable (by 10%), achievable (realistic improvement), relevant (improves cardiovascular fitness), and time-bound (three months).

Creating a personalized fitness plan based on your baseline assessments and goals is crucial for making consistent progress. Your plan should include a balanced mix of cardiovascular exercises, strength training, flexibility work, and rest days. For instance, if your baseline assessment revealed weak core strength, incorporating more core-focused exercises like planks, Russian twists, and leg raises into your routine would be beneficial.

Tracking your progress is just as important as setting a baseline. Regularly re-evaluating your fitness level using the same tests allows you to see improvements, stay motivated, and adjust your workouts as needed. Keeping a fitness journal or using a fitness app can help you record your workouts, track your progress, and celebrate milestones.

Consider the story of John, a 35-year-old who decided to improve his fitness after years of a sedentary lifestyle. John began by setting a baseline through various fitness tests. His 12-minute run test indicated poor cardiovascular endurance, and his push-up test showed below-average upper body strength. His flexibility tests revealed tight hamstrings and limited shoulder mobility. Using this information, John set specific goals: to increase his 12-

minute run distance by 15% in six months, double the number of push-ups he could perform, and improve his flexibility to touch his toes.

John created a fitness plan that included three days of cardiovascular exercise, two days of strength training, and daily stretching. He tracked his progress in a journal, noting improvements and any challenges he faced. After three months, he re-evaluated his fitness level and was pleased to see significant improvements in all areas. His run distance had increased by 10%, he could perform 50% more push-ups, and his flexibility had improved noticeably. These results motivated John to continue his fitness journey, setting new goals and adjusting his plan as needed.

John's story illustrates the power of setting a baseline and using it to guide your fitness journey. By understanding your starting point, you can set realistic goals, create an effective plan, and track your progress. This approach not only enhances your physical fitness but also boosts your confidence and motivation.

In conclusion, setting a baseline for progress is a vital step in any fitness journey. By assessing your cardiovascular endurance, muscular strength, flexibility, and body composition, you can create a comprehensive picture of your current fitness level. Using this information to set SMART goals and design a personalized fitness plan ensures that you make consistent progress and stay motivated. Regularly re-evaluating your fitness level allows you to track improvements, celebrate milestones, and adjust your workouts as needed. Embrace the process of setting a baseline and enjoy the journey towards a healthier, fitter you.

Chapter 2: The Science of Exercise

Types of Physical Activity

Physical activity comes in many forms, each offering unique benefits and contributing to overall health and fitness in different ways. Understanding the various types of physical activity can help you create a balanced and effective exercise routine tailored to your individual needs and goals. This chapter explores the main categories of physical activity, including aerobic exercise, strength training, flexibility exercises, balance activities, and recreational sports, providing a comprehensive overview of how each can enhance your physical well-being.

Aerobic exercise, often referred to as cardio, is any activity that increases your heart rate and breathing while improving the efficiency of your cardiovascular system. Activities like running, cycling, swimming, and brisk walking are all excellent examples of aerobic exercise. These activities help strengthen the heart and lungs, improve circulation, and boost overall endurance. Regular aerobic exercise is known to reduce the risk of chronic diseases such as heart disease, stroke, and diabetes. Moreover, it can aid in weight management and improve mental health by reducing symptoms of anxiety and depression.

Strength training, or resistance training, involves exercises that work your muscles by using resistance, such as weights, resistance bands, or your body weight. Common strength training exercises include squats, deadlifts, bench presses, push-ups, and pull-ups. This type of physical activity is crucial for building and maintaining muscle mass, which naturally declines with age. Increased muscle mass boosts metabolism, helps maintain healthy body weight, and supports joint health by reducing the risk of injury. Strength training also enhances bone density, reducing the risk of osteoporosis, particularly important as we age.

Flexibility exercises focus on stretching the muscles and improving the range of motion of the joints. Yoga and Pilates are popular forms of flexibility exercises that also incorporate elements of balance and strength. Regular stretching helps maintain muscle elasticity and joint mobility, which can prevent injuries and improve physical performance. Flexibility exercises are particularly beneficial for individuals who engage in repetitive movements or sit for prolonged periods, as they help counteract muscle stiffness and imbalances.

Balance activities are designed to improve stability and coordination, which are essential for daily activities and preventing falls, especially in older adults. Tai Chi, a form of martial arts that emphasizes slow and controlled movements, is an excellent balance activity that also promotes relaxation and mental clarity. Simple exercises like standing on one leg, heel-to-toe walking, and using balance boards can also enhance balance and coordination. Incorporating balance exercises into your routine can improve proprioception, the body's ability to sense its position in space, which is crucial for overall mobility and function.

Recreational sports provide a fun and social way to stay active while improving various aspects of physical fitness. Sports like soccer, basketball, tennis, and volleyball offer a combination of aerobic exercise, strength training, and balance activities. Engaging in recreational sports can enhance cardiovascular health, build muscle strength, improve coordination, and boost mental well-being through social interaction and the enjoyment of the game. Additionally, the competitive nature of sports can motivate individuals to push themselves harder and achieve higher levels of fitness.

To illustrate the benefits of incorporating various types of physical activity into your routine, consider the story of Maria, a 45-year-old office worker who decided to improve her fitness after experiencing chronic back pain and fatigue. Maria began by integrating brisk walking into her daily routine, which helped her build cardiovascular endurance and lose weight. She then added strength training exercises twice a week, focusing on her core and back muscles to alleviate her pain and improve posture. To enhance her flexibility, Maria joined a weekly yoga class, which also helped her manage stress and improve her mental well-being. Finally, Maria started playing tennis with friends on weekends, combining fun and social interaction with a full-body workout. Over time, Maria noticed significant improvements in her strength, flexibility, balance, and overall energy levels, demonstrating the benefits of a well-rounded exercise routine.

When creating your exercise plan, it's important to consider your fitness level, goals, and any physical limitations or health conditions. Start with activities you enjoy and gradually increase the intensity and variety as your fitness improves. Aim for at least 150 minutes of moderate-intensity aerobic exercise or 75 minutes of vigorous-intensity aerobic exercise per week, combined with muscle-strengthening activities on two or more days per week. Additionally, incorporate flexibility and balance exercises into your routine to ensure a comprehensive approach to fitness.

Variety in your exercise routine not only prevents boredom but also reduces the risk of overuse injuries by targeting different muscle groups and movement patterns. Cross-training, or engaging in various types of physical activities, can help you achieve balanced fitness and avoid plateaus in your progress. For example, alternating between running, cycling, and swimming for aerobic exercise can prevent repetitive strain on specific muscles and joints. Similarly, combining different strength training exercises, such as free weights, resistance bands, and bodyweight exercises, can ensure a well-rounded approach to muscle development.

Listening to your body and allowing adequate rest and recovery is also crucial for long-term success. Overtraining can lead to burnout, injuries, and decreased performance. Ensure you have rest days in your weekly routine and pay attention to any signs of fatigue or discomfort. Proper nutrition, hydration, and sleep are essential components of recovery and overall health, supporting your body's ability to perform and adapt to physical activity.

Incorporating mindfulness into your exercise routine can enhance the benefits of physical activity. Mindful movement practices, such as yoga and Tai Chi, emphasize the connection between the mind and body, promoting relaxation and mental clarity. Even during more intense workouts, paying attention to your breath, posture, and the sensations in your body can improve your focus and performance. Mindfulness can also help you stay present and fully enjoy the experience of physical activity, making it a more rewarding and sustainable part of your lifestyle.

In conclusion, understanding the different types of physical activity and how they contribute to overall health and fitness is essential for creating a balanced and effective exercise routine. Aerobic exercise, strength training, flexibility exercises, balance activities, and recreational sports each offer unique benefits that can enhance various aspects of physical well-being. By incorporating a variety of activities into your routine, setting realistic goals, and listening to your body, you can achieve and maintain optimal fitness while enjoying the process. Embrace the diversity of physical activity and discover the many ways it can enrich your life, both physically and mentally.

The Physiology of Exercise

The human body is an intricate machine designed for movement, and understanding the physiology of exercise can help you harness its full potential. When you engage in physical activity, a cascade of physiological responses occurs, affecting nearly every system in your body. This chapter delves into the key physiological changes that happen during exercise, including cardiovascular adaptations, respiratory efficiency, muscular responses, and metabolic processes, providing you with a comprehensive understanding of how your body works to support physical activity.

When you begin exercising, one of the first systems to respond is the cardiovascular system. Your heart rate increases almost immediately to pump more blood, and therefore more oxygen and nutrients, to the working muscles. This is facilitated by the sympathetic nervous system, which stimulates the heart to beat faster and stronger. The stroke volume, or the amount of blood ejected by the heart with each beat, also increases, allowing more blood to circulate through your body. Over time, with consistent training, your heart becomes more efficient. The left ventricle, responsible for pumping oxygenated blood to the rest of the body, enlarges and strengthens, enabling it to pump a greater volume of blood with each beat. This is why endurance athletes often have lower resting heart rates; their hearts are highly efficient at delivering oxygen to tissues.

Simultaneously, exercise demands a higher respiratory rate to meet the increased oxygen requirements. Your breathing becomes deeper and more rapid, enhancing the amount of oxygen taken in and carbon dioxide expelled. The capillaries surrounding the alveoli in your lungs expand, improving the exchange of gases. With regular aerobic training, the efficiency of your respiratory system improves. The muscles involved in breathing, such as the diaphragm and intercostal muscles, become stronger, and the overall capacity of your lungs increases. This allows for more effective oxygen uptake and utilization, which translates to better endurance and performance.

Muscular responses to exercise are equally fascinating. When you perform physical activity, your muscles contract and generate force through a process called the sliding filament theory. This involves the interaction of actin and myosin, the proteins within muscle fibers. Initially, your muscles rely on stored adenosine triphosphate (ATP) for energy. However, ATP stores are limited and must be replenished quickly through metabolic processes. For short bursts of activity, muscles rely on anaerobic metabolism, which generates ATP without oxygen but produces lactic acid as a byproduct. This can lead to the familiar burning sensation during intense exercise.

For sustained activities, your body shifts to aerobic metabolism, which uses oxygen to produce ATP from carbohydrates, fats, and, to a lesser extent, proteins. This process is more efficient and can sustain longer periods of exercise. Regular training enhances the muscles' ability to store and use glycogen (stored form of glucose) and increases the number of mitochondria, the powerhouses of cells where aerobic metabolism occurs. This adaptation allows for greater energy production and improved endurance.

Muscle hypertrophy, or growth, is a common goal of strength training. When you lift weights or perform resistance exercises, you create microscopic tears in the muscle fibers. The body repairs these tears by fusing the fibers, increasing their size and strength. This process, known as muscle protein synthesis, is influenced by factors such as the type of exercise, nutrition, and recovery. Consuming adequate protein and allowing sufficient rest are crucial for maximizing muscle growth and repair.

Exercise also induces significant changes in your metabolic processes. Metabolism encompasses all the chemical reactions that occur within your body to maintain life, including those that convert food into energy. During exercise, your metabolic rate increases to meet the energy demands of your muscles. This heightened metabolic state persists even after you finish exercising, a phenomenon known as excess post-exercise oxygen consumption (EPOC). EPOC represents the amount of oxygen required to restore your body to its resting state, including replenishing ATP and clearing lactic acid. High-intensity interval training (HIIT) is particularly effective at boosting EPOC, leading to greater calorie burn post-workout.

Hormonal responses play a critical role in the physiology of exercise. Physical activity triggers the release of various hormones that regulate energy production, muscle growth, and recovery. For example, adrenaline and noradrenaline, released by the adrenal glands, increase heart rate, blood pressure, and energy availability. Cortisol, often called the stress hormone, helps mobilize energy stores but can also promote muscle breakdown if levels remain elevated for prolonged periods. Growth hormone and testosterone are essential for muscle repair and growth. Regular exercise, especially resistance training, can enhance the production and sensitivity of these anabolic hormones, supporting muscle development and overall physical performance.

The benefits of exercise extend to the nervous system as well. Physical activity stimulates the release of neurotransmitters like endorphins, dopamine, and serotonin, which improve mood, reduce stress, and enhance cognitive function. The increased blood flow to the brain during exercise delivers more oxygen and nutrients, promoting neurogenesis, the formation of new neurons. This can improve memory, learning, and overall brain health. Studies have shown that regular physical activity is associated with a lower risk of neurodegenerative diseases such as Alzheimer's and Parkinson's.

One often overlooked aspect of exercise physiology is its impact on the immune system. Moderate exercise can boost immune function by promoting the circulation of immune cells, enhancing their ability to detect and combat pathogens. However, it's important to note that excessive or intense exercise without adequate recovery can suppress immune function, making you more susceptible to illness. Striking a balance between exercise intensity and recovery is key to maintaining a healthy immune system.

Hydration and electrolyte balance are crucial during exercise, especially in hot and humid conditions. As you exercise, your body temperature rises, and you sweat to cool down. Sweat contains water and electrolytes, such as sodium, potassium, and magnesium, which are vital for maintaining fluid balance, muscle function, and nerve transmission. Dehydration can impair performance and increase the risk of heat-related illnesses. Drinking water and consuming electrolyte-rich foods or beverages can help maintain hydration status and support optimal performance.

To illustrate the profound effects of exercise on the body, consider the story of Alex, a 30-year-old who decided to train for a marathon. Initially, Alex struggled with shortness of breath and muscle fatigue during runs. However, as he adhered to a structured training program, his cardiovascular and respiratory systems adapted. His resting heart rate decreased, his lung capacity increased, and his muscles became more efficient at utilizing oxygen and energy stores. Alex's metabolic rate improved, and he experienced the benefits of EPOC, which helped him manage his weight. The regular release of endorphins and other neurotransmitters elevated his mood and reduced stress, making him more resilient to the challenges of daily life. By race day, Alex felt stronger, faster, and more confident, a testament to the remarkable physiological transformations brought about by consistent exercise.

Understanding the physiology of exercise underscores the importance of incorporating regular physical activity into your life. Each workout triggers a complex interplay of systems and processes that enhance your overall health and performance. By appreciating how your body responds and adapts to exercise, you can make informed decisions about your fitness routine, optimize your training, and achieve your health and fitness goals. Embrace the science behind exercise and let it guide you towards a stronger, healthier, and more vibrant life.

How Exercise Affects the Body

Engaging in regular exercise brings a multitude of benefits, affecting almost every part of your body. From the moment you start moving, a series of complex physiological responses begin, enhancing your physical and mental health in profound ways. Understanding these effects can provide motivation and insight into how to optimize your workouts for maximum benefit.

When you begin exercising, your cardiovascular system is one of the first to respond. Your heart rate increases to pump more blood, and consequently more oxygen and nutrients, to your working muscles. This increase in cardiac output is driven by the sympathetic nervous system, which stimulates the heart to beat faster and stronger. Over time, consistent cardiovascular exercise can lead to adaptations such as a stronger heart muscle and an increased stroke volume, meaning the heart pumps more blood with each beat. This efficiency is why athletes often have lower resting heart rates; their hearts are adept at delivering oxygen to tissues even during periods of rest.

Simultaneously, your respiratory system ramps up its efforts. You start breathing more rapidly and deeply to meet the higher oxygen demands of your body. The alveoli in your lungs, where the exchange of oxygen and carbon dioxide occurs, become more efficient with regular exercise. The muscles that aid in breathing, like the diaphragm, grow stronger, enhancing your overall lung capacity and function. This is particularly beneficial for endurance activities, where sustained oxygen delivery is crucial for performance.

The skeletal muscles are direct beneficiaries of your physical activity. As you exercise, your muscles contract and generate force through the sliding filament theory, where actin and myosin filaments within muscle fibers slide past each other. Initially, muscles rely on stored adenosine triphosphate (ATP) for energy, but these stores are quickly depleted. To continue generating energy, your body then uses anaerobic metabolism, which does not require oxygen but produces lactic acid as a byproduct. This can lead to muscle fatigue and the familiar burning sensation during intense exercise.

For activities of longer duration, your body shifts to aerobic metabolism, which uses oxygen to produce ATP from carbohydrates, fats, and proteins. This process is more efficient and can sustain prolonged exercise. Regular training enhances your muscles' ability to store and use glycogen, the stored form of glucose, and increases the number of mitochondria, the energy powerhouses of cells. These adaptations allow for greater energy production and improved endurance.

Resistance training induces muscle hypertrophy, the increase in muscle size. When you lift weights or perform resistance exercises, you create microscopic tears in muscle fibers. The body repairs these tears by fusing the fibers, increasing their size and strength. This process is influenced by factors such as the type of exercise, nutrition, and recovery. Adequate protein intake and sufficient rest are essential for maximizing muscle growth and repair.

Exercise also significantly impacts your metabolic processes. Metabolism encompasses all chemical reactions in your body that maintain life, including those that convert food into energy. During exercise, your metabolic rate increases to meet the energy demands of your muscles. This elevated metabolic state continues even after you stop exercising, known as excess post-exercise oxygen consumption (EPOC). EPOC involves the body consuming more oxygen to restore itself to its resting state, replenish ATP stores, and clear lactic acid. High-intensity interval training (HIIT) is particularly effective at boosting EPOC, resulting in greater calorie burn post-workout.

Hormonal responses are critical to the physiological changes induced by exercise. Physical activity triggers the release of various hormones that regulate energy production, muscle growth, and recovery. For instance, adrenaline and noradrenaline increase heart rate, blood pressure, and energy availability. Cortisol helps mobilize energy stores but can promote muscle breakdown if levels remain elevated for too long. Growth hormone and testosterone are pivotal for muscle repair and growth. Regular exercise, especially strength training, can enhance the production and sensitivity of these anabolic hormones, supporting muscle development and overall physical performance.

Exercise benefits extend to the nervous system as well. Physical activity stimulates the release of neurotransmitters like endorphins, dopamine, and serotonin, which improve mood, reduce stress, and enhance cognitive function. The increased blood flow to the brain during exercise delivers more oxygen and nutrients, promoting neurogenesis, the creation of new neurons. This can improve memory, learning, and overall brain health. Regular physical activity is associated with a lower risk of neurodegenerative diseases such as Alzheimer's and Parkinson's.

The immune system also experiences positive effects from exercise. Moderate exercise can boost immune function by promoting the circulation of immune cells, enhancing their ability to detect and combat pathogens. However, it's important to note that excessive or intense exercise without adequate recovery can suppress immune function, increasing susceptibility to illness. Balancing exercise intensity and recovery is key to maintaining a healthy immune system.

Hydration and electrolyte balance are crucial during exercise, especially in hot and humid conditions. As you exercise, your body temperature rises, and you sweat to cool down. Sweat contains water and electrolytes like sodium, potassium, and magnesium, which are vital for fluid balance, muscle function, and nerve transmission. Dehydration can impair performance and increase the risk of heat-related illnesses. Drinking water and consuming electrolyte-rich foods or beverages can help maintain hydration status and support optimal performance.

Consider the story of Sarah, a 35-year-old who decided to start a fitness journey. Initially, Sarah found herself out of breath and fatigued after just a few minutes of running. However, with persistence and a structured training program, her cardiovascular and respiratory systems adapted. Her resting heart rate decreased, lung capacity increased, and her muscles became more efficient at utilizing oxygen and energy stores. Sarah's metabolic rate improved, and she experienced the benefits of EPOC, helping her manage her weight. The regular release of endorphins and other neurotransmitters elevated her mood and reduced stress, making her more resilient to daily challenges. By sticking with her program, Sarah became stronger, faster, and more confident, showcasing the transformative power of regular exercise.

Understanding how exercise affects your body underscores the importance of making physical activity a regular part of your life. Each workout triggers a complex interplay of systems and processes that enhance your overall health and performance. By appreciating how your body responds and adapts to exercise, you can make informed decisions about your fitness routine, optimize your training, and achieve your health and fitness goals. Embrace the science behind exercise and let it guide you towards a stronger, healthier, and more vibrant life.

The Role of Rest and Recovery

Rest and recovery are integral components of any effective fitness regimen, yet they are often overlooked in the pursuit of physical goals. While the actual workout is critical for pushing the body to its limits, it is during rest and recovery that the body repairs, rebuilds, and strengthens itself. Understanding the role of these processes can help optimize performance, prevent injuries, and enhance overall well-being.

When you engage in physical activity, especially intense exercise, you create microscopic damage to muscle fibers. This damage is a natural and necessary part of muscle growth. During rest, the body goes to work repairing these fibers through a process called muscle protein synthesis. This involves the fusion of muscle fibers to form new muscle protein strands, leading to increased muscle mass and strength. Without adequate rest, the body cannot effectively perform these repairs, resulting in diminished gains and increased risk of injury.

Sleep is perhaps the most critical component of rest and recovery. During sleep, the body releases growth hormone, which is essential for muscle repair and regeneration. Quality sleep also allows the brain to recover, improving cognitive function, mood, and overall mental health. Sleep deprivation, on the other hand, can lead to increased levels of cortisol, a stress hormone that can inhibit muscle growth and impair recovery. Ensuring 7-9 hours of quality sleep each night can significantly enhance recovery and overall performance.

Nutrition plays a vital role in the recovery process. Consuming adequate amounts of protein is essential for muscle repair. Protein provides the building blocks, or amino acids, necessary for muscle protein synthesis. Carbohydrates are also important as they replenish glycogen stores that are depleted during exercise. Glycogen is the primary fuel source for high-intensity training, and without sufficient carbohydrates, performance can suffer. Fats, while often overlooked, are crucial for hormone production and overall health. Including a balanced diet with a mix of protein, carbohydrates, and fats can support optimal recovery.

Hydration is another key factor in recovery. Water is involved in almost every bodily function, including the transportation of nutrients and the removal of waste products. Dehydration can impair muscle function and delay recovery. Electrolytes, such as sodium, potassium, and magnesium, are also important as they help maintain fluid balance and muscle function. Drinking water throughout the day and consuming electrolyte-rich foods or beverages can aid in the recovery process.

Active recovery, which involves low-intensity exercise, can also be beneficial. Activities such as walking, swimming, or yoga can increase blood flow to muscles, helping to flush out waste products and deliver oxygen and nutrients. This can reduce muscle soreness and stiffness, promoting quicker recovery. Active recovery days can be strategically placed between more intense workout sessions to allow the body to recover while still maintaining a level of physical activity.

Listening to your body is crucial in understanding its need for rest. Signs of overtraining include persistent fatigue, decreased performance, increased susceptibility to illness, and prolonged muscle soreness. Ignoring these signs can lead to more serious injuries and setbacks. Incorporating rest days into your training schedule can prevent overtraining and ensure that you can continue to progress without interruption.

Mental recovery is equally important as physical recovery. Exercise places stress not only on the body but also on the mind. Taking time to relax and engage in activities that promote mental well-being can enhance overall recovery. Techniques such as meditation, deep breathing, and mindfulness can reduce stress and improve focus and mental clarity. Ensuring that you have a balanced approach to both physical and mental recovery can lead to better performance and a healthier lifestyle.

Rest and recovery also play a significant role in injury prevention. Overuse injuries, such as tendonitis and stress fractures, are often the result of insufficient recovery. These injuries can sideline athletes for extended periods and can be prevented by allowing adequate time for rest and repair. Incorporating stretching and mobility exercises can also aid in recovery and prevent injuries by improving flexibility and range of motion.

Consider the experience of John, an avid runner who was consistently pushing himself to improve his times. Despite his dedication, he began to notice a decline in performance and an increase in fatigue. By consulting with a coach, John learned the importance of incorporating rest days and adjusting his nutrition to support recovery. He also started prioritizing sleep and using active recovery techniques. As a result, John not only improved his performance but also felt more energized and less prone to injury.

Massage therapy can be a beneficial addition to a recovery routine. Massage can increase blood flow, reduce muscle tension, and promote relaxation. This can help alleviate muscle soreness and improve range of motion. While professional massage can be highly effective, self-massage techniques using tools such as foam rollers and massage balls can also provide significant benefits.

Another important aspect of recovery is the use of recovery tools and technologies. Compression garments, for example, can help reduce muscle soreness and improve circulation. Cold therapy, such as ice baths, can reduce inflammation and speed up recovery. Heat therapy can relax muscles and improve blood flow. Understanding and utilizing these tools can enhance the recovery process and support overall performance.

The timing of recovery is also critical. Post-workout nutrition, often referred to as the "anabolic window," is a period immediately following exercise when the body is particularly receptive to nutrients. Consuming a combination of protein and carbohydrates within this window can maximize muscle protein synthesis and glycogen replenishment. While the exact length of the anabolic window is debated, aiming to consume a balanced meal or snack within an hour of training can support recovery.

Incorporating variety into your training program can also aid in recovery. Cross-training, or engaging in different types of physical activities, can prevent overuse injuries and reduce mental fatigue. For example, a runner might benefit from incorporating swimming or cycling into their routine. This not only provides physical rest for certain muscle groups but also keeps the training program interesting and engaging.

Understanding the role of rest and recovery is essential for anyone looking to improve their fitness and overall health. By prioritizing sleep, nutrition, hydration, active recovery, and mental well-being, you can enhance your body's ability to repair and grow stronger. Listening to your body and incorporating rest days into your training schedule can prevent injuries and ensure long-term success. Embrace the importance of recovery and let it guide you towards achieving your fitness goals in a sustainable and balanced way.

Common Exercise Myths and Facts

Exercise often comes with a plethora of advice, much of which is steeped in myth rather than fact. These misconceptions can hinder progress, cause frustration, and sometimes even lead to injury. Dispelling these myths and understanding the facts can help beginners navigate the world of fitness more successfully.

One of the most pervasive myths is that lifting weights will make you bulky. This belief, particularly common among women, stems from the fear of developing a bodybuilder physique. However, building significant muscle mass requires specific training, nutrition, and often a genetic predisposition. For most people, especially women, lifting weights will instead result in a toned, stronger, and leaner body. Strength training is crucial for boosting metabolism, enhancing bone density, and improving overall functional fitness.

Another common misconception is that you need to spend hours at the gym to see results. The truth is, quality trumps quantity. Effective workouts can be short and intense. High-Intensity Interval Training (HIIT), for example, can deliver substantial benefits in a fraction of the time compared to traditional steady-state cardio. These shorter, more intense workouts increase cardiovascular fitness, burn calories, and improve muscle tone efficiently.

The idea that spot reduction is possible is another widespread myth. Many people believe that by targeting specific areas with exercises, such as doing countless sit-ups to get rid of belly fat, they can selectively lose fat in those areas. In reality, fat loss occurs throughout the entire body and is largely influenced by genetics, diet, and overall activity levels. A balanced approach to exercise, including both cardiovascular and strength training, combined with a healthy diet, is the most effective way to reduce body fat.

Cardio is often viewed as the ultimate solution for weight loss, but the belief that it is the only or best method is misguided. While cardiovascular exercise is excellent for heart health and can help burn calories, strength training is equally important.

Building muscle increases resting metabolic rate, meaning you burn more calories even when not exercising. A combination of both cardio and strength training yields the best results for overall fitness and weight management.

Many people think that sweating a lot means you're getting a better workout. Sweat is simply the body's way of cooling itself, not an indicator of workout intensity. Factors such as temperature, humidity, and individual physiology affect how much you sweat. A good workout is determined by the effort and engagement of muscles, not by the amount of sweat produced.

The belief that you must stretch before exercising is another myth. While stretching is important, static stretching (holding a stretch for an extended period) before a workout can actually weaken performance by temporarily reducing muscle strength. Dynamic warm-ups, which involve moving the muscles through their range of motion, are more effective at preparing the body for exercise. Static stretching is best saved for post-workout when muscles are warm and more pliable.

There's also the myth that you need to exercise every day to stay fit. While consistency is key, rest and recovery are equally important. Muscles need time to repair and grow stronger after workouts. Overtraining can lead to fatigue, injury, and diminished performance. Incorporating rest days and listening to your body's signals is crucial for long-term fitness success.

Some believe that running is bad for your knees. While it's true that running can cause knee problems for some, it's not inherently bad for the knees. Proper running technique, appropriate footwear, and a balanced training program that includes strength training can mitigate the risk of injury. For many, running can actually strengthen the muscles around the knees and improve joint health.

The idea that more protein equals more muscle is a myth that can lead to overconsumption of protein supplements. While protein is essential for muscle repair and growth, the body can only utilize so much. Excessive protein intake does not translate to more muscle gain and can put strain on the kidneys. It's important to consume a balanced diet with adequate protein, carbohydrates, and fats to support overall health and fitness goals.

Another common misconception is that older adults should avoid strength training. On the contrary, strength training is incredibly beneficial for older adults. It helps maintain muscle mass, improves bone density, enhances balance, and reduces the risk of falls. Age-appropriate strength training programs can significantly improve quality of life and independence in older adults.

A prevalent myth is that you should not eat before working out. While it's true that eating a large meal right before exercise can cause discomfort, having a small, balanced snack can provide the necessary energy for a more effective workout. Carbohydrates are particularly important as they fuel exercise. Finding what works best for your body through trial and error is key.

The myth that you can turn fat into muscle is another misunderstanding. Fat and muscle are two distinct types of tissue; one cannot be converted into the other. Fat loss and muscle gain can occur simultaneously with a combination of diet and exercise, but the processes are separate. Reducing body fat through cardiovascular exercise and a healthy diet, while building muscle through strength training, are both essential for body composition changes.

Finally, the belief that you must feel sore after every workout to see progress is false. While some muscle soreness, known as delayed onset muscle soreness (DOMS), is common when starting a new exercise routine or increasing intensity, it is not a requirement for improvement. Consistent, progressive training without excessive soreness is a sign of effective and sustainable exercise.

Understanding the facts behind these common exercise myths can empower beginners to make informed decisions about their fitness journey. By focusing on evidence-based practices and listening to their bodies, individuals can achieve their goals more efficiently and enjoyably. Embracing a balanced approach to exercise, incorporating both cardio and strength training, prioritizing rest and nutrition, and debunking these myths will lead to sustainable and successful fitness outcomes.

Chapter 3: Creating a Personalized Fitness Plan

Identifying Your Fitness Goals

Setting out on a fitness journey without a clear destination is like embarking on a road trip without a map. Identifying your fitness goals is the crucial first step that will define your path, keep you motivated, and ultimately determine your success. These goals should be specific, measurable, attainable, relevant, and time-bound (SMART), providing a clear roadmap to guide your efforts.

Begin by reflecting on why you want to get fit. Is it to improve your health, lose weight, build muscle, enhance athletic performance, or simply feel better in your own skin? Your motivations will shape your goals and the strategies you employ to achieve them. Personal motivations vary greatly, and understanding your own can help maintain focus and commitment through the inevitable challenges.

Health-related goals are often at the top of many people's lists. If your primary aim is to improve overall health, consider what specific aspects are most important to you. Are you looking to lower your blood pressure, improve cardiovascular fitness, manage diabetes, or enhance mental health? Each of these objectives will require different approaches. For example, cardiovascular fitness might be improved through regular aerobic exercises like walking, running, or cycling, while managing diabetes could involve a combination of exercise and dietary changes.

Weight loss is a common goal for many. However, it's important to approach this goal in a healthy and sustainable manner. Rather than fixating on a specific number on the scale, focus on reducing body fat and increasing lean muscle mass. This approach not only improves aesthetics but also enhances metabolic health. Incorporating both cardiovascular exercises and strength training into your routine, along with a balanced diet, can help achieve this goal. Remember, gradual weight loss is more sustainable and healthier than rapid weight loss.

Building muscle is another popular fitness goal. Whether you aspire to have a bodybuilder's physique or simply want to tone up, muscle growth requires a combination of resistance training, proper nutrition, and adequate rest. Identify which muscle groups you want to focus on and design a workout plan that targets these areas. Progressive overload, which involves gradually increasing the weight or resistance in your exercises, is key to muscle growth. Protein intake is also crucial, as it provides the building blocks for muscle repair and growth.

Enhancing athletic performance is a goal for many sports enthusiasts. Whether you're a runner, swimmer, cyclist, or play team sports, improving performance often involves a mix of skill-specific training, strength conditioning, and endurance work. Set goals that are specific to your sport. For instance, a runner might aim to improve their 5k time, while a basketball player might focus on increasing their vertical jump. Tailored training plans that address these specific needs will be most effective.

Mental health benefits are increasingly recognized as a significant motivator for fitness. Regular physical activity is known to reduce symptoms of anxiety and depression, improve mood, and enhance cognitive function. If mental well-being is your primary goal, consider incorporating activities that you enjoy and look forward to. This could be anything from yoga and

Pilates to running and dancing. The key is consistency and finding joy in movement.

Once you have identified your primary fitness goals, break them down into smaller, actionable steps. This makes them less overwhelming and provides a sense of accomplishment as you achieve each milestone. For example, if your goal is to run a marathon, your smaller steps might include running a 5k, then a 10k, and gradually increasing your distance over time. Celebrate these small victories as they are indicators of your progress.

It's also important to set both short-term and long-term goals. Short-term goals might include weekly or monthly targets, such as going to the gym three times a week or increasing your squat weight by 10 pounds. Long-term goals, on the other hand, could be six months to a year or more into the future, such as completing a half-marathon or achieving a certain body fat percentage. Having both types of goals keeps you motivated and provides a clear vision of where you're headed.

Tracking your progress is essential for staying on course. Keep a workout journal or use fitness apps to log your activities, track your improvements, and adjust your goals as needed. This not only helps you stay accountable but also allows you to see how far you've come, which can be incredibly motivating. Regularly reviewing and adjusting your goals ensures they remain relevant and challenging.

Flexibility in your goals is also crucial. Life is unpredictable, and there will be times when you need to adjust your plans. Whether it's due to an injury, a busy period at work, or personal commitments, being able to adapt your goals ensures you stay on track in the long term. This might mean modifying your workout intensity, trying new activities, or temporarily shifting your focus to maintain balance.

Another important aspect of setting fitness goals is seeking support. Share your goals with friends, family, or a fitness community. Having a support system can provide encouragement, advice, and motivation. Consider working with a personal trainer or joining group fitness classes to gain professional guidance and a sense of camaraderie.

It's also beneficial to educate yourself about fitness and nutrition. Understanding the science behind exercise and diet can empower you to make informed decisions and optimize your efforts. There are countless resources available, from books and articles to online courses and workshops. Continuously learning and staying curious will keep your fitness journey engaging and effective.

Don't forget the importance of recovery in achieving your fitness goals. Adequate rest, proper nutrition, and techniques like stretching, foam rolling, and massage are vital for preventing injuries and ensuring your body can perform at its best. Overtraining can be counterproductive, leading to burnout and setbacks. Listen to your body and prioritize recovery as part of your overall plan.

Lastly, maintain a positive mindset. Fitness is a journey with ups and downs. There will be days when you feel unstoppable and others when motivation wanes. Remember why you started and keep your goals in sight. Celebrate your progress, no matter how small, and don't be too hard on yourself during setbacks. Resilience and perseverance are key to long-term success.

Identifying your fitness goals is the foundation of a successful fitness journey. By setting clear, realistic, and meaningful goals, breaking them down into manageable steps, tracking your progress, and maintaining flexibility, you can achieve lasting results. Embrace the process, seek support, and continually educate yourself to stay motivated and on track. With dedication and a positive mindset, your fitness goals are well within reach.

Choosing the Right Types of Exercise

Embarking on your fitness journey involves a myriad of choices, one of the most crucial being the types of exercises you incorporate into your routine. Selecting the right exercises can make the difference between a sustainable, enjoyable fitness regimen and one that feels like a chore. It's essential to consider your fitness goals, preferences, and physical condition when crafting your exercise plan.

Cardiovascular exercises, or cardio, are fundamental for improving heart health, increasing stamina, and burning calories. Activities such as running, cycling, swimming, and brisk walking elevate your heart rate and enhance cardiovascular endurance. For beginners, it's advisable to start with moderate-intensity cardio like walking or light jogging, gradually increasing intensity and duration as your fitness level improves. Variety is key to preventing boredom and ensuring that all muscle groups are engaged. Try mixing in different cardio activities to keep things interesting and challenging.

Strength training, also known as resistance training, is another critical component of a balanced exercise routine. This type of exercise focuses on building muscle mass, increasing strength, and enhancing bone density. Incorporating weight lifting, bodyweight exercises like push-ups and squats, and resistance band exercises can significantly improve overall muscle tone and metabolic rate. Beginners should start with lighter weights and focus on proper form to avoid injury. As you become more comfortable and confident, gradually increase the weights and resistance to continue challenging your muscles.

Flexibility exercises, often overlooked, are vital for maintaining a full range of motion in the joints, preventing injuries, and reducing muscle stiffness. Activities such as yoga, Pilates, and dedicated stretching routines enhance flexibility and promote relaxation. Incorporating flexibility exercises into your routine can improve posture, balance, and overall physical performance. For those new to flexibility training, starting with a basic yoga class or a simple stretching routine can be beneficial. Consistency is more important than intensity, so aim to include flexibility exercises in your regimen a few times a week.

High-Intensity Interval Training (HIIT) has gained popularity for its efficiency and effectiveness. HIIT involves short bursts of intense exercise followed by brief periods of rest or lower-intensity exercise. This approach can maximize calorie burn, improve cardiovascular fitness, and build muscle in a shorter amount of time compared to traditional steady-state cardio. HIIT can be adapted to various fitness levels by adjusting the intensity and duration of the intervals. For beginners, it's crucial to ensure proper warm-up and cool-down periods to prevent injury and allow the body to acclimate to this demanding workout style.

Functional training focuses on exercises that mimic everyday movements, improving overall strength, balance, and coordination. This type of training is particularly beneficial for enhancing daily activities and reducing the risk of injury. Exercises such as squats, lunges, and kettlebell swings are staples of functional training. These movements engage multiple muscle groups simultaneously, promoting efficient and practical strength. Beginners should concentrate on mastering the correct form and gradually increasing the complexity of the exercises.

Group fitness classes offer a social and motivational environment that can be particularly appealing for beginners. Classes such as Zumba, spin, and aerobics provide structured workouts led by instructors, which can be helpful for those who prefer guided exercise. The camaraderie and accountability of group settings can enhance motivation and make the workout experience more enjoyable. If you're new to exercise, participating in a variety of classes can help you discover what you enjoy most and what best aligns with your fitness goals.

Mind-body exercises, like tai chi and certain forms of yoga, emphasize the connection between mental and physical well-being. These practices improve balance, coordination, and mental focus while promoting relaxation and stress reduction. Incorporating mind-body exercises into your routine can complement more intense workouts, providing a holistic approach to fitness. Beginners might find these exercises less intimidating and a gentle introduction to regular physical activity.

Outdoor activities such as hiking, kayaking, and cycling offer a refreshing alternative to indoor workouts. Engaging with nature can enhance mental well-being and provide a change of scenery that keeps exercise enjoyable. These activities can also be social, involving friends or family, which adds an extra layer of motivation. For beginners, starting with shorter, less challenging outdoor activities and gradually increasing the intensity and duration can make these exercises more accessible and enjoyable.

Combining different types of exercises is crucial for achieving a well-rounded fitness routine. Each type of exercise offers unique benefits, and a varied approach ensures that you address all aspects of physical fitness. For example, pairing strength training with cardio can enhance both muscle development and cardiovascular health. Adding flexibility exercises ensures that your muscles remain supple and reduce the risk of injury. A balanced routine might include strength training two to three times a week, cardio sessions on alternate days, and flexibility exercises incorporated throughout the week.

Listening to your body is paramount when choosing the right types of exercise. Pay attention to how different activities affect your body and adjust accordingly. If an exercise causes pain or discomfort, it might be necessary to modify it or choose a different activity. Consulting with a fitness professional or a physical therapist can provide personalized guidance, especially if you have any pre-existing conditions or injuries.

Setting realistic and attainable goals is essential for maintaining motivation and tracking progress. Whether your aim is to lose weight, build muscle, improve stamina, or simply stay active, having clear objectives helps in selecting the appropriate types of exercise. Regularly reviewing and adjusting your goals ensures that your fitness plan remains relevant and challenging.

Finding enjoyment in your workouts is perhaps the most critical factor in sustaining a long-term fitness routine. Experiment with different types of exercise to discover what you love. Whether it's the rhythm of a dance class, the solitude of a morning run, or the challenge of lifting weights, enjoyment breeds consistency. The more you enjoy your activities, the more likely you are to stick with them.

Integrating rest and recovery into your exercise routine is also essential. Overtraining can lead to burnout and injuries, derailing your fitness journey. Ensure that you include rest days and listen to your body's signals. Adequate sleep, proper nutrition, and hydration are vital components of recovery that support your fitness efforts.

Choosing the right types of exercise involves a combination of understanding your goals, experimenting with different activities, and listening to your body. By incorporating a variety of exercises—cardio, strength training, flexibility, HIIT, functional training, group classes, mind-body exercises, and outdoor activities—you can create a balanced, enjoyable, and effective fitness routine. Consistency, enjoyment, and a holistic approach to fitness will guide you toward achieving your goals and maintaining a healthy, active lifestyle.

Structuring a Balanced Workout Routine

Creating a balanced workout routine is essential for achieving fitness goals, whether it's building strength, losing weight, or improving overall health. A well-rounded plan not only enhances physical capabilities but also ensures long-term sustainability and reduces the risk of injury. To structure an effective workout routine, one must consider the various components of fitness: cardiovascular endurance, strength, flexibility, and rest.

Begin by assessing your current fitness level and identifying clear, achievable goals. This foundational step sets the direction for your workout plan. Are you aiming to run a marathon, build muscle mass, or simply stay active? Goals can vary widely, and they should be specific, measurable, attainable, relevant, and time-bound (SMART).

Start with cardiovascular exercises, which are crucial for heart health, improving stamina, and burning calories. These activities can range from running, cycling, and swimming to dancing and brisk walking. For beginners, it's essential to ease into cardio with moderate-intensity exercises, gradually increasing the duration and intensity as endurance improves. Aim for at least 150 minutes of moderate-intensity or 75 minutes of high-intensity cardio per week, spread across several days. This approach not only boosts cardiovascular health but also aids in weight management and enhances mood through the release of endorphins.

Strength training is the next vital component of a balanced workout routine. This type of exercise helps build muscle, increase bone density, and boost metabolism. Incorporating exercises that target all major muscle groups ensures a comprehensive approach. Beginners should start with bodyweight exercises such as push-ups, squats, and lunges, gradually progressing to free weights and resistance machines. It's important to focus on proper form to prevent injuries. Typically, strength training should be done two to three times a week, with at least one rest day between sessions to allow muscles to recover and grow.

Flexibility exercises often take a backseat but are crucial for maintaining a full range of motion in your joints and preventing injuries. Incorporating activities like yoga, Pilates, or simple stretching routines can improve flexibility and reduce muscle stiffness. Stretching should be done after workouts when muscles are warm, holding each stretch for 15-30 seconds. Aim to include flexibility exercises in your routine at least two to three times a week. Improved flexibility not only enhances performance in other exercises but also contributes to better posture and reduced muscle tension.

In addition to these core components, integrating functional training into your routine can provide significant benefits. Functional exercises mimic everyday movements, improving overall strength, coordination, and balance. Exercises such as squats, lunges, and kettlebell swings are excellent examples. They engage multiple muscle groups simultaneously, promoting efficient and practical strength. Functional training can be particularly beneficial for older adults or those recovering from injuries, as it enhances the ability to perform daily activities with ease.

High-Intensity Interval Training (HIIT) can be a powerful addition to a balanced workout routine. HIIT involves short bursts of intense exercise followed by brief periods of rest or lower-intensity activity. This method is highly effective for burning calories, improving cardiovascular fitness, and building muscle in a relatively short amount of time. Beginners should start with shorter intervals and gradually increase the intensity and duration as fitness levels improve. It's essential to warm up before and cool down after HIIT sessions to prevent injuries and aid recovery.

Rest and recovery are often overlooked but are critical components of a balanced workout routine. Overtraining can lead to burnout, injuries, and plateauing progress. Ensure that you schedule regular rest days to allow your body to recover and repair. Active recovery activities such as light walking, stretching, or yoga can be beneficial on rest days. Adequate sleep, proper nutrition, and hydration also play significant roles in recovery and overall performance.

To maintain motivation and track progress, it's helpful to keep a workout journal. Documenting workouts, noting improvements, and reflecting on challenges can provide valuable insights and keep you accountable. Setting short-term goals and celebrating milestones can also boost motivation and make the fitness journey more enjoyable.

Variety is another key element in structuring a balanced workout routine. Mixing different types of exercises prevents boredom, ensures all muscle groups are engaged, and avoids overuse injuries. For example, you could alternate between cardio, strength training, and flexibility exercises throughout the week. Trying new activities, such as dance classes, rock climbing, or hiking, can keep the routine fresh and exciting.

Listening to your body is paramount. Pay attention to how different exercises make you feel and adjust accordingly. If you experience pain or discomfort, it might be necessary to modify the exercise or seek professional advice. Consulting with a fitness trainer or physical therapist can provide personalized guidance, especially if you have any pre-existing conditions or injuries.

Nutrition plays a crucial role in supporting a balanced workout routine. Consuming a well-rounded diet that includes a mix of carbohydrates, proteins, fats, vitamins, and minerals provides the energy and nutrients needed for exercise and recovery. Staying hydrated is equally important, as dehydration can impair performance and recovery. Consider consulting with a nutritionist to tailor your diet to your specific fitness goals and needs.

Creating a balanced workout routine involves a thoughtful combination of various types of exercises, adequate rest, and proper nutrition. By incorporating cardiovascular exercises, strength training, flexibility workouts, functional training, and HIIT, you can address all aspects of physical fitness. Regularly assessing your progress, maintaining motivation through variety, and listening to your body ensure that your fitness journey is both enjoyable and sustainable. Remember, the key to long-term success is consistency, so find activities you enjoy and make them a regular part of your lifestyle.

Importance of Progressive Overload

Progressive overload is the cornerstone of any effective fitness regimen. It's a principle that involves gradually increasing the stress placed on the body during exercise to stimulate muscle growth, strength, and endurance. The concept is simple but powerful: to make continual progress in your fitness journey, your body must be challenged with increasing intensity over time. This incremental approach ensures that muscles are consistently pushed beyond their comfort zones, leading to adaptation and improvement.

The origins of progressive overload can be traced back to ancient Greece, where the legendary wrestler Milo of Croton is said to have lifted a calf daily until it grew into a full-sized bull. This story, whether myth or reality, beautifully illustrates the essence of progressive overload. By gradually increasing the weight he carried, Milo's muscles adapted to the growing load, making him stronger over time.

To effectively implement progressive overload, one must understand its various components. These include increasing the weight lifted, the number of repetitions performed, the number of sets, the frequency of workouts, or reducing rest periods between sets. Each of these methods places additional stress on the muscles, encouraging growth and strength increases.

For beginners, it's crucial to start with manageable weights and focus on proper form and technique. As you become more comfortable and your strength improves, you can begin to increase the weight gradually. A common approach is the 2-for-2 rule: if you can perform two more repetitions than your target in the last set of an exercise for two consecutive workouts, it's time to increase the weight. This method ensures that the increase in load is manageable and reduces the risk of injury.

Another effective way to apply progressive overload is by increasing the number of repetitions. For example, if you're performing three sets of 10 repetitions of a particular exercise, aim to add one or two repetitions each week. Once you can perform 15 repetitions with good form, it's time to increase the weight and start the process again. This method is particularly useful for beginners, as it allows the body to adapt gradually to increased demands.

Increasing the number of sets is another strategy. If you typically perform three sets of an exercise, try adding an additional set. This increases the overall volume of work your muscles are subjected to, promoting growth and endurance. However, it's essential to listen to your body and avoid overtraining. Recovery is a critical aspect of progressive overload, and muscles need time to repair and grow stronger between workouts.

Reducing rest periods between sets can also enhance progressive overload. Shortening the rest time forces your muscles to work harder, improving endurance and cardiovascular fitness. For instance, if you usually rest for 90 seconds between sets, try reducing it to 60 seconds. This approach can be particularly challenging and should be done gradually to prevent excessive fatigue and potential injury.

Frequency of workouts is another variable that can be adjusted. Increasing the number of workouts per week can lead to greater gains, provided that adequate recovery time is allowed. For example, if you currently train three times a week, adding an extra session can boost your progress. However, it's important to monitor your body's response and ensure that this increased frequency does not lead to overtraining.

Progressive overload is not limited to weight lifting. It applies to all forms of exercise, including cardiovascular training. Runners can increase their mileage or pace gradually to improve endurance and speed. Cyclists can add more challenging routes or increase their ride duration. Swimmers can increase the number of laps or reduce rest intervals. The key is to consistently challenge your body to adapt to greater demands.

Tracking your progress is essential for effectively implementing progressive overload. Keeping a workout log can help you monitor the weights, repetitions, sets, and rest periods for each exercise. This record allows you to see your improvements over time and adjust your plan accordingly. It also provides motivation as you reflect on how far you've come.

Listening to your body is paramount when applying progressive overload. While the goal is to challenge yourself, it's important to distinguish between good pain (muscle fatigue and soreness) and bad pain (sharp or persistent discomfort that could indicate injury). If you experience the latter, it's crucial to rest and seek professional advice if necessary. Pushing through pain can lead to serious injuries and setbacks.

Nutrition plays a significant role in supporting progressive overload. Adequate protein intake is essential for muscle repair and growth. Carbohydrates provide the energy needed for intense workouts, while healthy fats support overall health and hormone production. Staying hydrated is also crucial, as dehydration can impair performance and recovery.

Rest and recovery are critical components of progressive overload. Muscles grow and strengthen during rest periods, not during the workout itself. Ensuring you get enough sleep, incorporating rest days into your routine, and considering activities like yoga or light stretching can aid recovery. Overtraining can lead to burnout, injuries, and diminished progress, so it's essential to balance hard work with adequate rest.

Mental fortitude is often overlooked but is a crucial aspect of applying progressive overload. Challenging workouts require mental strength and resilience. Setting short-term goals, celebrating small victories, and maintaining a positive mindset can help you stay motivated. Visualization techniques and positive self-talk can also enhance performance and keep you focused on your long-term objectives.

As you progress in your fitness journey, it's important to periodically reassess and adjust your goals. What worked in the beginning may need modification as you become stronger and more conditioned. Regularly evaluating your progress and setting new challenges ensures that you continue to improve and avoid plateaus.

Progressive overload is a fundamental principle for anyone looking to improve their fitness level. By gradually increasing the demands placed on your body, you stimulate muscle growth, enhance strength, and boost endurance. Whether through increasing weights, repetitions, sets, frequency, or reducing rest periods, consistently challenging your body leads to continual progress. Remember to track your progress, listen to your body, support your efforts with proper nutrition and recovery, and maintain mental resilience. Through a thoughtful and disciplined approach to progressive overload, you can achieve your fitness goals and enjoy long-term success.

Adapting Your Plan Over Time

Fitness journeys are dynamic, requiring flexibility and adaptability to achieve long-term success. As you progress, your body and mind will experience changes, necessitating adjustments to your workout plan. Adapting your plan over time ensures that you continue to make gains, avoid plateaus, and keep your routine fresh and engaging.

One of the first signals that it's time to adapt your plan is when you hit a plateau. Plateaus occur when your body becomes accustomed to the stress you place on it, leading to stagnation in progress. This can be frustrating, but it's an opportunity to reassess and modify your workout regimen. Changing variables such as exercise type, intensity, duration, and frequency can help break through these plateaus.

Variety is essential in a fitness plan. Repeating the same exercises can lead to boredom and decreased motivation. More importantly, your muscles adapt to familiar routines, reducing their effectiveness. To keep your workouts challenging and engaging, regularly incorporate new exercises that target the same muscle groups but in different ways. For example, if you usually perform barbell squats, try incorporating goblet squats or Bulgarian split squats. These variations not only keep things interesting but also target muscles from different angles, promoting balanced development.

Progressive overload is another crucial element in adapting your plan. As your strength and endurance improve, gradually increasing the intensity of your workouts is necessary. This can be achieved by adding more weight, increasing the number of repetitions or sets, or reducing rest intervals. For instance, if you've been comfortably lifting a certain weight for several weeks, it might be time to increase the load. Similarly, if your endurance training has become easier, consider extending the duration or intensity of your sessions.

Listening to your body is vital when adapting your fitness plan. Signs of overtraining, such as prolonged muscle soreness, fatigue, and decreased performance, indicate the need for rest or a change in your routine. Incorporating rest days and active recovery, such as light stretching or yoga, can help prevent burnout and injuries. Sometimes, scaling back on intensity or frequency for a period allows your body to recover, leading to better long-term results.

Setting new goals is an integral part of adapting your plan. As you achieve your initial objectives, it's important to establish new ones to maintain motivation and progress. These goals can be more challenging or focus on different aspects of fitness. For example, if you've reached your weight loss target, you might shift your focus to building muscle or improving cardiovascular endurance. Setting SMART (specific, measurable, attainable, relevant, time-bound) goals helps provide direction and keeps you motivated.

Tracking your progress is essential for effective adaptation. Keeping a workout journal or using fitness apps allows you to monitor improvements and identify areas needing adjustment. Documenting details such as weights lifted, distances run, and times achieved provides a clear picture of your progress and helps in making informed changes to your plan. Regularly reviewing your progress ensures that you stay on track and make necessary adjustments to continue moving forward.

Nutrition is another critical aspect that may need adaptation over time. As your fitness level and goals evolve, so do your nutritional requirements. If your goal shifts from weight loss to muscle gain, you might need to increase your protein and calorie intake. Conversely, if you're focusing on endurance, you may require more carbohydrates to fuel your workouts. Consulting with a nutritionist can help tailor your diet to your changing needs, ensuring you get the right balance of macronutrients and micronutrients to support your goals.

Mental and emotional factors also play a significant role in adapting your plan. As your fitness journey progresses, you might encounter periods of low motivation or mental fatigue. Incorporating variety and setting new challenges can help keep your workouts exciting and mentally stimulating. Additionally, finding a workout buddy or joining a fitness community can provide social support and accountability, making it easier to stay committed.

Periodization is a strategic approach to adapting your plan. This method involves cycling through different phases of training, each with specific goals and focus areas. For example, you might spend several weeks building muscle (hypertrophy phase), followed by a strength phase, and then a phase focused on endurance or functional fitness. Periodization helps prevent overtraining, reduces the risk of injury, and ensures balanced development across different fitness components.

Functional training is another aspect to consider when adapting your plan. Functional exercises mimic everyday movements, improving overall strength, coordination, and balance. Incorporating exercises like kettlebell swings, medicine ball throws, and stability ball exercises can enhance your functional fitness, making daily activities easier and reducing the risk of injury. This approach is particularly beneficial as you age or if you have specific physical demands in your daily life or occupation.

Flexibility and mobility exercises should also be integrated into your evolving fitness plan. As you increase the intensity and variety of your workouts, ensuring your muscles and joints can handle the new demands is crucial. Incorporating regular stretching, yoga, or Pilates sessions can improve flexibility, enhance performance, and reduce the risk of injury. These practices also promote relaxation and recovery, contributing to overall well-being.

Adapting your plan over time also involves paying attention to the recovery process. As you progress, your body's recovery needs may change. Implementing techniques such as foam rolling, massage, and adequate sleep can aid in faster recovery and better performance. Additionally, as you increase the intensity of your workouts, ensuring you have sufficient rest days becomes even more important to allow your muscles to repair and grow.

Listening to feedback from your body and making data-driven decisions is crucial. Wearable fitness technology, such as heart rate monitors and activity trackers, can provide valuable insights into your performance and recovery. By analyzing this data, you can make informed adjustments to your plan, ensuring you continue to make progress without risking overtraining or injury.

Adapting your fitness plan over time is essential for sustained progress and long-term success. Incorporating variety, progressively increasing intensity, setting new goals, and listening to your body are key strategies for effective adaptation. Tracking progress, adjusting nutrition, considering mental and emotional factors, and implementing periodization and functional training all contribute to a well-rounded and dynamic fitness plan. By staying flexible and responsive to your body's needs, you can continue to make gains, avoid plateaus, and maintain a fulfilling and enjoyable fitness journey.

Chapter 4: Nutrition and Fitness

Basic Nutrition Principles

Nutrition plays a fundamental role in achieving and maintaining optimal health, especially when combined with a consistent fitness regimen. Understanding basic nutrition principles can empower you to make informed choices that support your fitness goals and overall well-being. Let's delve into the essential components of a balanced diet, the importance of macronutrients and micronutrients, and practical strategies for eating healthier.

Macronutrients are the nutrients your body needs in large amounts: carbohydrates, proteins, and fats. Each serves a unique and vital function. Carbohydrates are your body's primary energy source. They are broken down into glucose, which fuels your brain and muscles during exercise. Complex carbohydrates, found in whole grains, vegetables, and legumes, provide sustained energy and are rich in fiber, aiding digestion and satiety. Simple carbohydrates, such as those in fruits and refined sugars, offer quick energy but should be consumed in moderation to avoid spikes in blood sugar levels.

Proteins are the building blocks of your body. They are crucial for repairing and building muscle tissues, producing enzymes and hormones, and supporting immune function. High-quality protein sources include lean meats, fish, eggs, dairy products, legumes, and plant-based proteins like tofu and quinoa. Aim to include a variety of protein sources in your diet to ensure you get all the essential amino acids your body needs for optimal functioning.

Fats, often misunderstood, are essential for health. They provide energy, support cell growth, protect your organs, and help your body absorb vitamins. There are different types of fats: unsaturated fats (found in olive oil, nuts, and avocados) are beneficial and should be included in your diet, while saturated and trans fats (found in fried foods, processed snacks, and some animal products) should be limited. Balancing your fat intake is key to maintaining heart health and overall wellness.

Micronutrients, though needed in smaller amounts, are equally important. These include vitamins and minerals that support various bodily functions such as metabolism, bone health, and immune response. Vitamins like A, C, D, E, and K, along with B-complex vitamins, play critical roles in maintaining health. Minerals such as calcium, potassium, magnesium, and iron are vital for bone strength, muscle function, and oxygen transport. A diet rich in fruits, vegetables, whole grains, and lean proteins usually provides adequate amounts of these essential nutrients.

Hydration is another crucial aspect of nutrition. Water is essential for every cell in your body, helping to regulate temperature, transport nutrients, and remove waste. Dehydration can impair physical performance, cognitive function, and overall health. Aim to drink at least eight 8-ounce glasses of water a day, more if you are physically active or live in a hot climate. Listen to your body's signals and drink when you feel thirsty, but also be proactive about maintaining hydration throughout the day.

Balancing your diet involves more than just nutrient intake; it also includes meal timing and portion control. Eating regular, balanced meals helps maintain energy levels and prevents overeating. Breakfast, often dubbed the most important meal of the day, kickstarts your metabolism and provides the energy needed for morning activities. Lunch and dinner should include a mix of macronutrients to sustain energy and support muscle recovery. Healthy snacks, such as fruits, nuts, and yogurt, can help keep hunger at bay and provide additional nutrients.

Portion control is vital for managing calorie intake and maintaining a healthy weight. Understanding serving sizes and listening to your body's hunger and fullness cues can prevent overeating. Using smaller plates, measuring portions, and being mindful of what you eat can help control portions. It's easy to overeat when not paying attention, especially with calorie-dense foods like snacks and desserts.

Mindful eating is a practice that can transform your relationship with food. It involves paying full attention to the eating experience, savoring each bite, and listening to your body's hunger and satiety signals. This approach can help you make healthier food choices, enjoy your meals more, and prevent overeating. Instead of eating in front of the TV or while on the go, try to take time to sit down and appreciate your food.

Understanding food labels is another practical skill. Labels provide information on serving sizes, calories, and nutrient content, helping you make informed choices. Pay attention to the ingredients list, aiming for foods with whole, unprocessed ingredients. Watch for added sugars, unhealthy fats, and high sodium levels, which can contribute to chronic health issues if consumed in excess.

Meal planning and preparation can also support healthier eating habits. Planning your meals in advance can save time, reduce stress, and ensure you have nutritious options available.

Preparing meals at home allows you to control the ingredients and portion sizes. Batch cooking and using leftovers creatively can make healthy eating more convenient and less time-consuming.

Supplements can be useful in certain situations but should not replace a balanced diet. They can fill nutritional gaps, especially if you have specific deficiencies or dietary restrictions. However, it's important to choose high-quality supplements and consult with a healthcare provider before starting any new supplement regimen. Over-reliance on supplements can lead to imbalances and potential health risks.

Special dietary needs and preferences, such as vegetarianism, veganism, gluten-free diets, or food allergies, require careful planning to ensure nutritional adequacy. Each of these diets can be healthy if well-planned to include a variety of nutrient-dense foods. For instance, vegetarians and vegans should focus on getting enough protein from plant sources, as well as essential nutrients like vitamin B12, iron, and omega-3 fatty acids, which are typically found in animal products.

Cultural and personal preferences also play a role in nutrition. Enjoying a wide variety of foods from different cultures can enhance your diet and make eating more enjoyable. Be open to trying new foods and recipes, and adapt traditional dishes to make them healthier without sacrificing flavor.

Finally, maintaining a healthy relationship with food is crucial. Food should be seen as fuel and nourishment, not as a reward or punishment. Avoid restrictive diets that can lead to unhealthy eating patterns and focus on balance and moderation. Emotional eating, often triggered by stress or boredom, can be managed by finding alternative coping strategies, such as physical activity, hobbies, or talking to a friend.

Nutrition is a complex but essential aspect of health and fitness. By understanding the roles of macronutrients and micronutrients, staying hydrated, practicing mindful eating, and adopting balanced meal planning, you can support your fitness goals and overall well-being. Embrace variety, listen to your body, and make informed choices to create a sustainable and enjoyable nutrition plan that complements your lifestyle and enhances your health.

Macronutrients and Their Role in Fitness

Macronutrients are the foundation of any effective fitness plan, each playing a critical role in fueling your body, building muscle, and supporting overall health. Understanding how carbohydrates, proteins, and fats contribute to your fitness goals can help you tailor your diet to maximize performance and recovery. Let's explore the unique functions of each macronutrient and how to effectively incorporate them into your diet.

Carbohydrates are often considered the primary energy source for active individuals. They are broken down into glucose, which is used by your muscles and brain for fuel. During exercise, especially high-intensity or endurance activities, your body relies heavily on stored glycogen, derived from carbohydrates, to maintain performance. Complex carbohydrates, such as those found in whole grains, vegetables, and legumes, provide a steady release of energy, helping to sustain prolonged physical activity.

Simple carbohydrates, like those in fruits and some processed foods, offer quick energy but should be consumed in moderation to avoid unwanted spikes in blood sugar levels.

A runner preparing for a marathon might prioritize carb-loading in the days leading up to the race. This strategy involves increasing carbohydrate intake to maximize glycogen stores in the muscles, ensuring ample energy reserves for the long run. Similarly, athletes involved in sports requiring quick bursts of energy, like basketball or soccer, benefit from a diet rich in carbohydrates to maintain peak performance throughout their games.

Proteins are the building blocks of muscle and are crucial for repair and growth. After a strenuous workout, your muscles undergo microscopic tears that need to be repaired. This is where protein plays its vital role, helping to rebuild and strengthen muscle fibers. High-quality protein sources include lean meats, fish, eggs, dairy products, and plant-based options like beans, lentils, and quinoa. For those engaged in regular strength training, it's important to consume adequate protein to support muscle hypertrophy and recovery.

Imagine a weightlifter who follows a rigorous training schedule. To maximize muscle gain and recovery, they might consume protein-rich meals and snacks throughout the day. Post-workout nutrition often includes a combination of protein and carbohydrates to replenish glycogen stores and kickstart the muscle repair process. For instance, a smoothie made with Greek yogurt, berries, and spinach provides a balanced mix of nutrients to support recovery.

Fats, though often misunderstood, are essential for overall health and play a key role in fitness. They provide a concentrated source of energy, support cell structure, and aid in the absorption of fat-soluble vitamins like A, D, E, and K. Unsaturated fats, found in foods like avocados, nuts, seeds, and olive oil, are beneficial and should be included in a balanced diet. Saturated fats, present in animal products and some processed foods, should be consumed in moderation to maintain heart health.

Endurance athletes, such as long-distance cyclists, often rely on fats for sustained energy, especially during prolonged activities where glycogen stores may deplete. Incorporating healthy fats into meals can help provide the necessary energy and improve overall performance. For example, a cyclist might add almond butter to their morning oatmeal or have a handful of nuts as a pre-ride snack to ensure they have a steady energy supply.

Balancing macronutrient intake is crucial for optimizing fitness outcomes. The right proportions depend on individual goals, activity levels, and metabolic rates. A balanced diet typically consists of approximately 45-65% of calories from carbohydrates, 10-35% from protein, and 20-35% from fats. However, these ratios can be adjusted based on specific needs. For instance, a bodybuilder aiming to increase muscle mass might increase their protein intake, while an endurance athlete might prioritize carbohydrates for sustained energy.

Meal timing and composition also play a significant role in maximizing the benefits of macronutrients. Consuming a balanced meal with a mix of carbohydrates, proteins, and fats before exercise can provide the energy needed for performance. Post-exercise nutrition is equally important for recovery, with a focus on replenishing glycogen stores and providing protein for muscle repair. A well-timed meal or snack can enhance recovery and prepare the body for the next workout session.

Consider a triathlete who plans their meals around training sessions. Before a long swim, they might have a breakfast rich in complex carbohydrates and moderate protein, such as oatmeal with almond butter and a banana. Post-swim, they could opt for a protein shake with added greens and a piece of whole-grain toast to replenish energy and aid in muscle recovery.

Hydration, while not a macronutrient, is another critical aspect of nutrition that affects fitness. Water is essential for maintaining bodily functions, regulating temperature, and supporting overall performance. Dehydration can impair physical abilities, leading to fatigue and decreased coordination. It's important to drink water regularly throughout the day and increase intake during and after exercise to replace fluids lost through sweat.

A practical approach to hydration involves drinking water before, during, and after workouts. For example, a runner might start their day with a glass of water, carry a water bottle during their run, and rehydrate with an electrolyte-rich drink post-run. This strategy helps maintain hydration levels and supports optimal performance.

Supplements can complement a balanced diet, particularly for those with specific needs or dietary restrictions. Protein supplements, such as whey or plant-based powders, can help meet protein requirements, especially for those with high training volumes. However, it's important to prioritize whole foods and use supplements as an adjunct rather than a replacement for a nutritious diet.

A busy professional who trains in the early morning might find it challenging to prepare a full meal post-workout. In such cases, a protein shake with added fruits and vegetables can provide a convenient and nutrient-dense option to support recovery until they can have a more substantial meal.

Special dietary considerations, such as vegetarianism, veganism, or food allergies, require careful planning to ensure adequate macronutrient intake. Plant-based diets can provide all necessary macronutrients when diverse and well-balanced. For instance, combining different plant proteins, such as beans and rice, can provide a complete amino acid profile, supporting muscle repair and growth.

A vegan athlete might focus on incorporating a variety of plant-based protein sources, such as tofu, tempeh, lentils, and chia seeds, to meet their protein needs. They might also pay attention to their intake of healthy fats by including foods like avocados, nuts, and seeds in their diet. Ensuring a well-rounded intake of all macronutrients supports their training and overall health.

Ultimately, understanding macronutrients and their roles in fitness can empower you to make informed dietary choices that enhance performance, recovery, and overall well-being. By balancing carbohydrates, proteins, and fats, and considering individual needs and goals, you can create a nutrition plan that supports your fitness journey. Embrace variety, prioritize whole foods, and listen to your body's signals to optimize your nutrition and achieve your fitness aspirations.

Pre- and Post-Workout Nutrition

Fueling your body correctly before and after workouts is crucial to maximizing performance, enhancing recovery, and achieving your fitness goals. Pre- and post-workout nutrition not only provides the necessary energy for exercise but also helps in muscle repair and growth. Understanding what to eat and when can make a significant difference, whether you're a beginner or a seasoned athlete.

Imagine you're about to embark on a morning run or an intense gym session. What you eat before this activity can set the tone for your entire workout. Consuming a balanced meal or snack that includes carbohydrates, proteins, and fats can provide sustained energy and prevent fatigue. Carbohydrates are particularly important pre-workout because they quickly convert to glucose, the primary energy source for your muscles. Opt for complex carbs like oatmeal, whole-grain bread, or sweet potatoes, which release energy slowly and keep your blood sugar levels stable.

A common pre-workout meal might include a bowl of oatmeal topped with a banana and a dollop of almond butter. The oatmeal provides complex carbs, the banana offers quick-digesting sugars and potassium, and the almond butter adds healthy fats and a bit of protein. This combination ensures a steady energy supply and helps prevent muscle cramps.

Proteins play a supportive role in pre-workout nutrition by providing amino acids that help in muscle maintenance and reduce muscle breakdown during exercise. Including a moderate amount of protein in your pre-workout meal can be beneficial, but it's important to avoid heavy, high-fat foods that might slow digestion and cause discomfort. A small serving of Greek yogurt with berries or a smoothie made with protein powder, spinach, and a few slices of fruit can be effective options.

Hydration is another critical aspect of pre-workout preparation. Dehydration can lead to decreased performance, increased heart rate, and a higher risk of injury. Drinking water throughout the day and consuming about 16-20 ounces of water an hour before your workout can help ensure you're well-hydrated. For longer or more intense workouts, you might also consider beverages with electrolytes to maintain proper fluid balance.

As you complete your workout, your muscles are in a state of repair and recovery. What you consume post-workout can significantly impact how well and how quickly you recover. The goal of post-workout nutrition is to replenish glycogen stores, repair muscle protein, and rehydrate. Timing is crucial; consuming a meal or snack within 30 minutes to two hours after your workout can maximize the benefits.

Carbohydrates are essential post-workout to restore the glycogen that your muscles have used up during exercise. The amount needed can vary based on the intensity and duration of your workout. Endurance athletes might require more carbs compared to someone who did a light workout. Simple carbs like fruits, white rice, or a sports drink can be beneficial immediately after a workout for quick glycogen replenishment.

Protein is vital post-workout to aid in muscle repair and growth. Aim for high-quality protein sources that provide all essential amino acids. The quantity can vary, but a general recommendation is to consume 20-40 grams of protein post-workout. This can come from sources like lean meats, fish, eggs, dairy products, or plant-based proteins like tofu or legumes.

A balanced post-workout meal might include grilled chicken breast, a serving of brown rice, and a side of steamed vegetables. This meal offers a combination of protein to repair muscles, carbohydrates to replenish glycogen, and vitamins and minerals to support overall recovery.

Fat intake post-workout is less critical but still important. Healthy fats can help reduce inflammation and support overall recovery. Including a small amount of fat in your post-workout meal, such as olive oil in a salad or a few slices of avocado, can be beneficial without slowing down digestion.

Hydration post-workout is just as important as pre-workout. Replenishing the fluids lost through sweat can prevent dehydration and support recovery. Drinking water or an electrolyte beverage can help restore fluid balance. Monitoring the color of your urine can be a simple way to ensure you're adequately hydrated; pale yellow indicates good hydration, while darker urine suggests you need more fluids.

Supplements can also play a role in pre- and post-workout nutrition, though they should complement a well-balanced diet rather than replace whole foods. Pre-workout supplements often contain ingredients like caffeine, beta-alanine, and branched-chain amino acids (BCAAs) that can enhance performance and reduce fatigue. Post-workout supplements, such as whey protein powder or creatine, can support muscle repair and growth.

Consider an athlete who uses a pre-workout supplement containing caffeine and BCAAs before a high-intensity training session. The caffeine can improve focus and endurance, while the BCAAs can help reduce muscle soreness. After the workout, they might consume a protein shake with whey protein and a banana to quickly provide the necessary nutrients for recovery.

Special dietary needs and preferences, such as veganism or gluten intolerance, require careful planning to ensure adequate pre- and post-workout nutrition. Plant-based athletes can obtain necessary nutrients from sources like quinoa, lentils, tofu, and a variety of fruits and vegetables. For instance, a vegan might have a smoothie made with plant-based protein powder, spinach, and berries before a workout and a meal of quinoa salad with chickpeas and vegetables afterward.

Listening to your body's signals is crucial in determining what works best for you. Everyone's nutritional needs and responses to food can vary. Paying attention to how different foods affect your energy levels and recovery can help you fine-tune your pre- and post-workout nutrition. Keeping a food and workout journal can be a helpful tool in tracking what works best for your body.

Ultimately, effective pre- and post-workout nutrition is about providing your body with the right nutrients at the right times to support your fitness goals. By focusing on balanced meals and snacks, staying hydrated, and listening to your body's needs, you can enhance your performance, speed up recovery, and achieve better results from your workouts. Whether you're preparing for a marathon, lifting weights, or engaging in a yoga session, the right nutrition can make a significant difference in how you feel and perform.

Hydration Strategies

Water is the essence of life, and nowhere is this more evident than in athletic performance and daily fitness activities. Proper hydration strategies can significantly influence how you feel, perform, and recover from exercise. Whether you're a weekend warrior, a seasoned runner, or someone just starting their fitness journey, understanding the principles of effective hydration is crucial.

Imagine stepping onto the track for a morning run. The sun is just peeking over the horizon, and the air is crisp and fresh. You're ready to conquer your miles, but have you considered how hydrated you are? The amount of water you drink can dramatically impact your endurance and overall experience. Dehydration, even at mild levels, can lead to decreased performance, increased perception of effort, and greater risk of heat-related illnesses.

Water is the most vital nutrient for athletes, and it's essential to start your day well-hydrated. Drinking a glass of water first thing in the morning helps replenish fluids lost overnight. Throughout the day, aim to drink regularly rather than waiting until you feel thirsty. Thirst is a late indicator of dehydration, and by the time you feel it, your performance may already be compromised.

A practical approach to maintaining hydration is to monitor the color of your urine. Pale yellow urine typically indicates adequate hydration, while darker shades suggest you need more fluids. This simple, non-invasive method can be an excellent guide to ensure you're drinking enough.

Before a workout, it's important to pre-hydrate. Consuming about 16-20 ounces of water two to three hours before exercising can help ensure your body is ready for the physical demands ahead. Additionally, drinking another 8-10 ounces about 20-30 minutes before you start can top off your hydration levels. This strategy helps prevent dehydration and can enhance your performance, especially in hot and humid conditions.

During exercise, fluid loss through sweat can be substantial, particularly in high-intensity or long-duration activities. It's critical to replace these lost fluids to maintain performance and prevent heat-related issues. A general guideline is to drink 7-10 ounces of water every 10-20 minutes during exercise. However, individual needs can vary based on factors like sweat rate, exercise intensity, and environmental conditions.

For those engaging in prolonged or intense exercise, water alone might not be sufficient. This is where sports drinks containing electrolytes like sodium, potassium, and magnesium come into play. Electrolytes help maintain fluid balance, support nerve function, and prevent muscle cramps. Consuming a sports drink during extended workouts can help replace electrolytes lost through sweat and provide carbohydrates for additional energy.

Consider an endurance runner tackling a marathon. Throughout the race, they might alternate between water and an electrolyte beverage at aid stations. This approach helps maintain hydration levels and ensures a steady supply of essential minerals that are crucial for muscle function and overall performance.

Post-exercise hydration is just as important as pre- and during-exercise strategies. Rehydrating after a workout helps in recovery, replenishes fluids lost through sweat, and can reduce muscle soreness. Weighing yourself before and after exercise can give you an idea of how much fluid you need to replace. For every pound lost during a workout, aim to drink about 16-24 ounces of water.

Including electrolytes in your post-workout hydration can also be beneficial. This can be achieved through sports drinks or natural sources like a banana or a handful of nuts. These foods provide not only electrolytes but also other nutrients that support recovery.

Hydration isn't just about what you drink during workouts; it's a 24/7 commitment. Your daily fluid intake should support your overall activity level and help maintain optimal hydration. The "8x8" rule—eight 8-ounce glasses of water a day—is a good starting point, but individual needs vary. Factors such as body size, activity level, and climate all influence how much water you need.

For example, someone living in a hot, humid climate or engaging in intense physical activity will require more fluids than someone living in a cooler environment or leading a sedentary lifestyle. Listening to your body and adjusting your fluid intake accordingly is key.

While water is the best choice for staying hydrated, other beverages can also contribute to your daily fluid needs. Herbal teas, milk, and even some fruits and vegetables with high water content, like cucumbers and watermelon, can help keep you hydrated. However, it's important to be mindful of beverages that can contribute to dehydration, such as those containing caffeine or alcohol. These should be consumed in moderation, especially around workout times.

Hydration strategies also extend to special situations like travel, altitude, or illness. Traveling, especially by air, can be dehydrating due to the low humidity in airplane cabins. Drinking water regularly during flights and avoiding excessive caffeine and alcohol can help mitigate this effect. At high altitudes, the body loses water more rapidly due to increased breathing rates and dry air, so staying vigilant about fluid intake is crucial.

Illnesses that cause fever, vomiting, or diarrhea can also lead to significant fluid loss. In such cases, oral rehydration solutions or electrolyte-rich beverages can help restore balance and prevent dehydration.

Finally, it's worth noting that overhydration, or hyponatremia, can be as dangerous as dehydration. This condition occurs when the balance of electrolytes in your body is disrupted by excessive water intake, leading to symptoms like nausea, headache, and in severe cases, seizures or coma. It's important to strike a balance and not overconsume water, particularly during endurance events.

Consider the case of a novice runner training for their first half-marathon. They might diligently follow hydration guidelines but overdo it by drinking large amounts of water without accounting for electrolyte balance. This could lead to hyponatremia, underscoring the importance of understanding and applying hydration strategies appropriately.

In summary, effective hydration strategies are multifaceted and personalized. They involve pre-hydration, maintaining fluid balance during exercise, and rehydrating post-exercise, all while considering individual needs and environmental factors. By paying attention to your body's signals and making hydration a priority, you can enhance your performance, support recovery, and achieve your fitness goals with greater ease and comfort.

Chapter 5: Making Smart Exercise Choices

Cardio vs. Strength Training

Cardio and strength training are two pillars of a well-rounded fitness regimen, each offering unique benefits and playing distinct roles in achieving overall health and fitness goals. Understanding the differences, benefits, and how to effectively incorporate both into your routine can help you maximize your workout efficiency and enjoy a balanced, healthy lifestyle.

Cardio, short for cardiovascular exercise, involves activities that increase your heart rate and improve the efficiency of your cardiovascular system. Common forms of cardio include running, cycling, swimming, and aerobics. These activities are often rhythmic and sustained over a period, making your heart and lungs work harder to pump blood and oxygen throughout your body.

Imagine a runner lacing up their shoes for a morning jog. As they set off, their heart rate begins to rise, and their breathing deepens. This process strengthens the heart muscle, increases lung capacity, and promotes better circulation. Over time, regular cardio exercise can lower the risk of heart disease, improve cholesterol levels, and enhance overall cardiovascular health.

Strength training, on the other hand, focuses on building muscle mass, strength, and endurance. This type of exercise involves resistance, whether through free weights, machines, or bodyweight exercises like push-ups and squats. Strength training causes microscopic damage to muscle fibers, which then repair and grow stronger during recovery.

Picture someone lifting weights at the gym. Each repetition challenges their muscles, creating tiny tears that the body will repair, making the muscles stronger and more resilient. This process not only builds physical strength but also boosts metabolism, supports bone health, and improves posture and balance.

Both cardio and strength training offer significant health benefits, but they serve different purposes and should be integrated thoughtfully into your fitness routine. Cardio is particularly effective for burning calories and improving cardiovascular health. It's ideal for those looking to lose weight or maintain a healthy weight, as it creates a calorie deficit by increasing energy expenditure.

Consider a cyclist pedaling through the countryside. The steady, rhythmic motion burns calories efficiently, helping to shed excess weight. Over time, this can lead to a leaner body composition and improved overall fitness.

In contrast, strength training is essential for building and maintaining muscle mass, which naturally declines with age. Incorporating strength exercises into your routine can help counteract this loss, preserving muscle function and metabolic rate. Increased muscle mass also means your body burns more calories at rest, contributing to long-term weight management.

Think of someone performing a series of squats and lunges. As they build muscle in their legs and core, they're not only enhancing their physical strength but also boosting their metabolism. This dual benefit makes strength training a critical component of any fitness program.

Balancing cardio and strength training in your routine can be challenging, but it's crucial for achieving a well-rounded fitness profile. The key is to find a balance that aligns with your personal fitness goals, whether that's weight loss, muscle gain, improved endurance, or overall health.

For beginners, starting with moderate-intensity cardio exercises like brisk walking or light jogging can build a foundation of cardiovascular fitness. Aim for at least 150 minutes of moderate-intensity or 75 minutes of high-intensity cardio per week, as recommended by health guidelines. This can be broken down into manageable sessions, such as 30 minutes five times a week.

As your endurance improves, you can incorporate more vigorous activities like running, cycling, or HIIT (high-intensity interval training). HIIT, in particular, is highly effective as it alternates between short bursts of intense activity and periods of rest or lower-intensity exercise, maximizing calorie burn and cardiovascular benefits in a shorter time.

Strength training should be added to your routine at least two to three times a week, targeting all major muscle groups. Beginners might start with bodyweight exercises such as push-ups, squats, and planks, gradually progressing to free weights or resistance machines as they build strength and confidence.

Imagine someone new to fitness starting with a simple routine: three sets of 10 squats, push-ups, and lunges, performed twice a week. As they become more comfortable, they might add dumbbells to increase resistance or incorporate additional exercises like deadlifts and bench presses.

It's also essential to allow time for recovery between strength training sessions, as muscles need time to repair and grow stronger. This doesn't mean you have to rest completely; light cardio or flexibility exercises like yoga can be excellent on non-strength training days.

Combining cardio and strength training in a single workout session can also be effective. For example, you might start with a 20-minute cardio warm-up, followed by 30 minutes of strength training. This approach ensures you're getting the benefits of both types of exercise without having to dedicate separate sessions to each.

Listening to your body and adjusting your routine based on how you feel is crucial. Overtraining can lead to fatigue, injury, and burnout, so it's important to find a sustainable balance that allows for consistent progress without overextending yourself.

Think of an athlete who balances their training by alternating between cardio and strength days, ensuring they get the benefits of both while minimizing the risk of injury. This strategic approach allows them to train consistently, improve performance, and stay motivated.

Nutrition and hydration are also vital components of an effective fitness regimen. Proper fuel before and after workouts can enhance performance and recovery. Carbohydrates provide energy for cardio sessions, while protein supports muscle repair and growth after strength training. Staying hydrated helps maintain performance and aids in recovery by preventing dehydration and muscle cramps.

Consider someone preparing for a workout by having a balanced meal that includes complex carbohydrates, lean protein, and healthy fats. Post-workout, they might have a protein shake or a meal rich in protein and carbs to support muscle recovery and replenish energy stores.

Ultimately, the most effective fitness routine is one that combines the strengths of both cardio and strength training, tailored to your individual goals and preferences. By integrating both types of exercise, you can enjoy the benefits of improved cardiovascular health, increased muscle mass, better weight management, and overall enhanced physical fitness.

Personalizing your approach and staying consistent are key to long-term success. Whether you're running through the park, lifting weights at the gym, or doing a mix of both, finding enjoyment in your activities will keep you motivated and committed to your fitness journey.

High-Intensity Interval Training (HIIT)

High-Intensity Interval Training (HIIT) has revolutionized the fitness world with its efficient and effective approach to exercise. HIIT involves alternating short bursts of intense activity with periods of lower intensity or rest, making it a time-efficient way to improve cardiovascular fitness, burn calories, and build muscle. This chapter delves into the principles of HIIT, its benefits, and how to incorporate it into your fitness routine effectively.

Imagine a busy professional struggling to find time for a workout. Traditional exercise routines might require an hour or more, but HIIT can deliver significant benefits in much less time. A typical

HIIT session might last anywhere from 15 to 30 minutes, making it an ideal choice for those with tight schedules. The secret lies in the intensity and the structured intervals that push your body to work harder, followed by recovery periods that prepare you for the next burst.

One of the primary benefits of HIIT is its impact on cardiovascular health. During high-intensity intervals, your heart rate spikes, and your cardiovascular system works intensely to supply oxygen to your muscles. Over time, this can lead to improvements in cardiac output and oxygen utilization, enhancing overall cardiovascular performance. Studies have shown that HIIT can be as effective, if not more so, than traditional moderate-intensity continuous training (MICT) in improving cardiovascular health.

Consider a scenario where you sprint for 30 seconds, followed by a 90-second walk or slow jog. This cycle repeats for 20 minutes. The intense sprints challenge your heart and lungs, while the recovery periods prevent complete exhaustion, allowing you to sustain the workout for the entire duration. Over time, this not only improves your endurance but also boosts your anaerobic capacity, which is crucial for high-intensity activities.

HIIT is also renowned for its efficiency in burning calories and promoting weight loss. The high-intensity bursts elevate your metabolic rate, not just during the workout, but for hours afterward—a phenomenon known as excess post-exercise oxygen consumption (EPOC). This means your body continues to burn calories even after the workout has ended, making HIIT a powerful tool for weight management.

Picture an individual performing a series of burpees, push-ups, and jump squats in rapid succession. Each exercise pushes their body to its limit, creating a significant calorie burn. Once the workout is over, their metabolism remains elevated as the body recovers and repairs, contributing to additional calorie expenditure. This afterburn effect is a key advantage of HIIT, making it highly effective for those looking to lose weight or maintain a lean physique.

In addition to cardiovascular and metabolic benefits, HIIT can also enhance muscle strength and endurance. While traditional strength training focuses on lifting heavy weights with longer rest periods, HIIT incorporates bodyweight exercises or lighter weights with minimal rest, creating a different type of muscular challenge. This approach can lead to improvements in muscular endurance and functional strength, benefiting everyday activities and sports performance.

Imagine a HIIT circuit that includes exercises like kettlebell swings, lunges, and mountain climbers. Each move targets different muscle groups, and the high-intensity nature of the workout ensures that your muscles are working hard. Over time, this can lead to increased muscle tone and strength, even without heavy lifting. The variety of exercises also keeps the workouts engaging and challenging, reducing the risk of boredom and plateau.

HIIT is highly adaptable and can be modified to suit different fitness levels and goals. Beginners might start with a simple routine, such as alternating between 30 seconds of fast walking and 30 seconds of slow walking. As fitness improves, the intensity and complexity of the exercises can be increased. Advanced HIIT routines might include sprinting, plyometric exercises, or advanced bodyweight moves, pushing the body to its limits.

Consider someone new to fitness who begins with a low-impact HIIT session. They might alternate between marching in place and light jogging. As they become more comfortable and their fitness level increases, they progress to exercises like jumping jacks, high knees, and eventually, sprint intervals. This gradual progression ensures that they are continuously challenged, leading to steady improvements in fitness and performance.

Safety is a critical consideration when incorporating HIIT into your routine. The high-intensity nature of the workouts can increase the risk of injury, particularly for those new to exercise or with underlying health conditions. It's essential to start slowly and focus on proper form, gradually increasing the intensity and complexity of the exercises. Listening to your body and allowing adequate recovery time between sessions can also help prevent overtraining and injury.

Imagine an athlete pushing themselves too hard during a HIIT session, neglecting proper form in their eagerness to complete the workout. This could lead to strains or sprains, setting back their fitness progress. By prioritizing form and allowing for rest, they can ensure that their workouts are both effective and safe, paving the way for long-term success.

In addition to physical benefits, HIIT can also have a positive impact on mental health. The intense nature of the workouts requires focus and determination, providing a mental challenge that can build resilience and reduce stress. The release of endorphins during high-intensity exercise can also boost mood and promote a sense of well-being, making HIIT a valuable component of a holistic approach to health.

Consider someone going through a stressful period who turns to HIIT as a way to cope. The physical exertion and mental focus required during the workout provide a temporary escape from their worries. The endorphin rush that follows leaves them feeling more positive and energized, ready to tackle their challenges with renewed vigor.

To incorporate HIIT into your fitness routine, start by identifying your goals and current fitness level. Beginners might aim for two to three HIIT sessions per week, gradually increasing the duration and intensity as their fitness improves. More advanced individuals might incorporate HIIT into their routine four to five times a week, ensuring that they vary the exercises to target different muscle groups and prevent overuse injuries.

Imagine a weekly workout plan that includes a mix of HIIT, strength training, and rest days. On HIIT days, you might focus on different types of exercises, such as running intervals, bodyweight circuits, or plyometric drills. Strength training days could involve traditional weightlifting or resistance exercises, while rest days allow for recovery and regeneration. This balanced approach ensures that all aspects of fitness are addressed, leading to comprehensive improvements in health and performance.

In conclusion, High-Intensity Interval Training (HIIT) offers a time-efficient, effective way to improve cardiovascular health, burn calories, and build muscle. Its adaptability makes it suitable for all fitness levels, and its benefits extend beyond physical health to mental well-being. By incorporating HIIT into your routine, you can achieve your fitness goals more efficiently and enjoy a balanced, healthy lifestyle.

Low-Impact Exercise Options

Low-impact exercise options offer a versatile and accessible means to stay fit, particularly for those who have joint issues, are recovering from injuries, or are new to fitness. These exercises minimize the stress placed on your joints and are ideal for maintaining cardiovascular health, improving flexibility, and building strength without the high risk of injury associated with high-impact activities.

Consider water aerobics, an excellent low-impact exercise that provides resistance training and cardiovascular benefits. The buoyancy of the water supports your body, reducing the stress on your joints while still offering a challenging workout. For example, someone with arthritis might find that walking or jogging in a pool allows them to exercise without exacerbating their joint pain. The natural resistance of the water helps to tone muscles and improve cardiovascular health, making it a full-body workout.

Swimming is another aquatic exercise that is gentle on the joints while providing a robust cardiovascular workout. The rhythmic nature of swimming can also have a meditative effect, reducing stress and improving mental well-being. Imagine gliding through the water, your body supported and your movements smooth and fluid. This can be particularly beneficial for those who find traditional forms of exercise uncomfortable or painful.

Walking is perhaps the most accessible form of low-impact exercise and can be easily incorporated into daily routines. A brisk walk in a park not only boosts cardiovascular health but also provides an opportunity to enjoy nature, which can enhance mental clarity and reduce stress. Picture a morning routine where you lace up your sneakers and head out for a 30-minute walk. The fresh air and rhythmic pace can set a positive tone for the rest of your day.

Cycling, whether on a stationary bike or outdoors, is another low-impact option that can be adjusted to various fitness levels. Stationary bikes are particularly useful as they allow for controlled, consistent movement and are gentler on the knees compared to running. A beginner might start with short sessions at a comfortable pace, gradually increasing the duration and intensity as their fitness improves. Outdoor cycling adds the element of navigating different terrains, which can increase the workout's challenge and keep it engaging.

Yoga, with its focus on flexibility, strength, and mindfulness, is an excellent low-impact exercise. Different styles of yoga can cater to varying fitness levels and goals. Hatha yoga, for instance, is gentle and suitable for beginners, emphasizing basic postures and breathing techniques. Imagine a sequence of poses that stretch and strengthen muscles while promoting relaxation and stress relief. Over time, regular practice can lead to improved flexibility, balance, and overall physical and mental well-being.

Pilates, similar to yoga, emphasizes core strength, flexibility, and controlled movement. It is particularly effective for improving posture and developing a strong, balanced body. Picture a Pilates session where you engage your core muscles to perform slow, deliberate movements. This focus on precision and control makes Pilates an ideal choice for those looking to enhance their overall physical condition without high-impact stress on their joints.

Elliptical machines provide a low-impact cardiovascular workout that can be adjusted for intensity and resistance. Unlike running on a treadmill, using an elliptical reduces the impact on your knees and hips while still offering a vigorous workout. Envision a workout where you glide smoothly on the elliptical, your legs moving in a natural, low-impact pattern. This can be particularly beneficial for those recovering from lower-body injuries or looking to avoid high-impact activities.

Tai Chi, an ancient Chinese martial art, combines slow, deliberate movements with deep breathing and meditation. It is often described as "meditation in motion" and is particularly beneficial for improving balance, flexibility, and mental focus. Imagine a group practicing Tai Chi in a tranquil park, their movements synchronized and graceful. This form of exercise is especially advantageous for older adults or those with chronic conditions, as it promotes physical health and mental tranquility without placing undue stress on the body.

Strength training can also be adapted to a low-impact format by using resistance bands or light weights. These tools allow for controlled, low-impact movements that build muscle strength and endurance. For instance, a beginner might use resistance bands to perform bicep curls, squats, or shoulder presses. The resistance bands provide a steady, controlled level of tension, reducing the risk of injury and making strength training accessible to those who might find traditional weight lifting too strenuous.

Dance-based workouts, such as Zumba or ballroom dancing, offer a fun and engaging way to improve cardiovascular fitness and coordination without high impact. These classes often incorporate a variety of movements that can be modified to suit different fitness levels. Picture a lively Zumba class with participants of all ages moving to the rhythm of upbeat music. The social aspect of group dance classes can also enhance motivation and make exercise feel less like a chore and more like a social activity.

Rowing, whether on a machine or in a boat, provides a full-body workout that is low-impact yet highly effective. The rowing motion engages multiple muscle groups, including the legs, core, and upper body, while the seated position reduces stress on the joints. Imagine rowing on a calm lake, each stroke propelling you smoothly across the water. This type of exercise can be particularly appealing for those looking for a comprehensive workout that is gentle on the body.

It's essential to start any new exercise routine slowly and listen to your body, especially if you are new to fitness or have existing health concerns. Consulting with a healthcare provider or fitness professional can help tailor a low-impact exercise plan that meets your individual needs and goals. They can provide guidance on proper form, progression, and how to incorporate variety to keep the workouts challenging and enjoyable.

Incorporating low-impact exercises into your routine can provide numerous health benefits without the high risk of injury. These exercises can improve cardiovascular health, build strength and flexibility, and enhance mental well-being. By choosing activities that you enjoy and that fit your lifestyle, you are more likely to stick with your exercise routine and achieve long-term health and fitness goals. Whether it's a brisk walk in the park, a refreshing swim, or a calming yoga session, low-impact exercises offer a sustainable path to a healthier, more active life.

Functional Fitness and Everyday Activities

Functional fitness focuses on exercises that train your muscles to work together and prepare them for daily tasks by simulating common movements you might do at home, work, or in sports. These exercises emphasize core stability and strength training that can help you perform everyday activities more easily and without injury. Incorporating functional fitness into your routine can enhance your ability to perform tasks such as lifting groceries, climbing stairs, or playing with your children.

Consider the act of lifting a heavy box from the floor. This movement relies on a combination of squats and deadlifts, which engage your core, legs, and back. By training these muscles through functional fitness exercises, you can improve your strength and reduce the risk of injury. For example, a squat mimics the motion of sitting down and standing up, which is a fundamental movement in daily life. Practicing squats with proper form can enhance your ability to perform this action with ease and safety.

Balancing exercises are another crucial aspect of functional fitness. Good balance is essential for preventing falls and maintaining agility in your daily activities. Simple exercises like standing on one leg or using a balance board can significantly improve your stability. Imagine standing on one leg while brushing your teeth or waiting in line; this small practice can make a considerable difference in your balance over time.

Core strength is at the heart of functional fitness. A strong core supports your spine and aids in nearly every movement you make. Exercises such as planks, Russian twists, and bicycle crunches target your core muscles, building the strength needed for activities ranging from bending to tie your shoes to maintaining proper posture while sitting at a desk. Picture yourself carrying a heavy bag of groceries; a strong core helps you stabilize and carry the load more effectively, reducing strain on your back.

Incorporating lunges into your fitness routine can also benefit your daily movements. Lunges mimic the action of stepping forward to reach for something or climbing stairs. By practicing lunges, you strengthen your legs, hips, and core, making these everyday actions more manageable. Visualize reaching to pick up a laundry basket from the floor; a strong, stable lunge form makes this task easier and safer.

Functional fitness also includes exercises that improve your range of motion and flexibility. Stretching and mobility exercises like yoga or dynamic stretches prepare your body for various movements and reduce the risk of injury. For instance, stretching your hamstrings can make it easier to bend down and reach under a table or into a low cabinet. Imagine starting your day with a few gentle yoga poses that open up your hips and shoulders, setting a positive tone for your body and mind.

Incorporating resistance training with free weights or resistance bands can further enhance your functional fitness. These tools allow you to perform compound movements that engage multiple muscle groups simultaneously. For example, a bicep curl combined with a squat targets your arms, legs, and core all at once. This type of functional training not only builds strength but also improves coordination and balance. Picture yourself lifting a child or a heavy suitcase; the strength and coordination gained from resistance training make these tasks feel less daunting.

Functional fitness can be seamlessly integrated into your daily routine without requiring a gym membership or special equipment. Simple activities such as gardening, playing with your kids, or even cleaning the house can be turned into functional exercises. Think about the movement patterns involved in raking leaves or scrubbing the floor; these actions require bending, lifting, and twisting, which are all fundamental functional movements. By being mindful of your body mechanics during these activities, you can turn everyday chores into effective workouts.

Practicing functional fitness can also enhance your athletic performance. Sports often require a combination of strength, agility, and endurance, all of which can be improved through functional training. For example, if you enjoy playing tennis, incorporating lateral lunges and rotational exercises into your routine can improve your side-to-side movement and power during swings. Visualize yourself on the tennis court, moving more efficiently and powerfully due to your functional training.

One of the key benefits of functional fitness is its adaptability. Regardless of your age or fitness level, you can modify functional exercises to suit your needs. For older adults, functional fitness can improve balance and mobility, reducing the risk of falls. For someone recovering from an injury, gentle functional movements can aid in rehabilitation and prevent further injury. Imagine an elderly person who regularly practices functional fitness; their improved balance and strength allow them to navigate stairs and uneven surfaces more confidently.

To get started with functional fitness, focus on compound movements that mimic your daily activities. Begin with bodyweight exercises such as squats, lunges, and planks, gradually adding resistance as you build strength. Pay attention to proper form to maximize the benefits and minimize the risk of injury. Envision a workout routine that includes a variety of movements, each targeting different muscle groups and simulating common tasks you perform every day.

Consistency is key to seeing improvements in functional fitness. Aim to incorporate functional exercises into your routine at least two to three times a week. Over time, you'll notice increased strength, better balance, and an overall improvement in your ability to perform everyday tasks. Think about the long-term benefits of this type of training; not only will you feel stronger and more capable, but you'll also reduce your risk of injury and improve your quality of life.

Functional fitness is a practical and effective approach to improving your overall health and well-being. By focusing on movements that enhance your ability to perform everyday activities, you can build strength, improve balance, and increase flexibility. Whether you're lifting groceries, playing sports, or simply going about your daily routine, functional fitness prepares your body to handle the demands of life with greater ease and confidence. Embrace the principles of functional fitness and discover how it can transform your daily movements into opportunities for improved health and vitality.

9 798330 331598